Straight Talk about ADHD in Girls

How to Help Your Daughter Thrive

Stephen P. Hinshaw, PhD

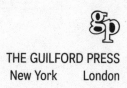

THE GUILFORD PRESS
New York   London

Published by The Guilford Press
A Division of Guilford Publications, Inc.
370 Seventh Avenue, Suite 1200, New York, NY 10001
www.guilford.com

Printed in the United States of America

This book is printed on acid-free paper.

Last digit is print number: 9   8   7   6   5   4   3   2   1

Library of Congress Cataloging-in-Publication Data is available from the publisher.

ISBN 978-1-4625-4751-7 (paperback) — ISBN 978-1-4625-4969-6 (hardcover)

Contents

Preface

Here's why I decided to write this book: Mainly because ADHD in girls is a most important and often neglected topic. A great number of parents and families out there are suffering from a lack of accurate information and helpful advice. So are their daughters. If you are a parent of a girl who has been diagnosed with ADHD, or if you believe she might have ADHD, you want her to thrive, just as you want any of your children to thrive. My goal is to give you the best possible chance of making that happen.

Throughout my career I have worked with and investigated children and adolescents with a range of neurodevelopmental and emotional conditions, particularly ADHD. I'm interested not only in the biological (including genetic) underpinnings of such disorders but also the treatments with the best evidence for helping affected individuals, the settings and contexts in which affected individuals can best thrive, and the potential for turning high-risk situations into resilient functioning.

Years ago, as a graduate student, I learned that ADHD (then called "hyperactivity"), and conditions like it, were the province of boys. I had my doubts, but there was little in the way of research evidence to support my views. Then, as a professor, having conducted a number of relevant studies, I finally got up the courage to write a grant to the National Institute of Mental Health to examine, as systematically as possible, whether girls with ADHD actually existed. The aim was to investigate the particular issues and problems they would encounter in naturalistic research summer programs, parallel to the ones I'd been conducting with boys for many years. Overall, the goal was to examine participants not in a pristine laboratory setting but in the kinds of contexts mirroring their everyday interactions. The additional hope was that we could follow our participants well beyond childhood.

Once the initial grant was funded and our team began our investigation, it quickly became clear that there was a huge need to understand the realities of ADHD in girls. There were many more girls than we could accept at our programs. At the same time I was involved with a large multicenter clinical trial of optimal treatments for boys and girls with ADHD (called the Multimodal Treatment Study of Children with ADHD). This additional participation furthered my interest in optimal treatments, including combinations of psychosocial and medication interventions, that could yield important clinical outcomes.

With the initial success of both studies, our respective teams were able to secure subsequent funding to follow the participants and their families into adolescence and emerging adulthood. In these unprecedented investigations, we have learned that ADHD is far from a transient condition in girls—and that families require abundant information, and support, to maintain the daily struggle to work with their daughters to promote thriving. In short, ADHD is truly a girl thing and not just a guy thing.

Over the ensuing years, I have also taken on the topic of the stigma that, tragically, still clings to a range of mental and neurodevelopmental disorders, including ADHD. The roots of this interest lie in my own family. Many of my family members have experienced serious mental illness and neurodevelopmental conditions, while at the same time encountering strong pressures (even from mental health professionals) to keep these problems completely hidden from view. I lived my own childhood in enforced silence about my father's extraordinarily severe (and misdiagnosed) bipolar disorder, wondering whether it was actually my fault that he vanished for months, or as much as a year at a time, into some of the country's worst mental institutions. He barely survived some of these stays because of the brutal "treatment" he received. I have also witnessed a range of other conditions—depression, ADHD, eating disorders, schizophrenia, substance abuse—in additional family members. I have had my own share of depressions.

As a result, during college and beyond, I resolved to devote my career to conducting programs for youth with neurodevelopmental and mental conditions, to better understand the causes and developmental course of such disorders, to treat them effectively, and to reduce the stigma that still too often stops the conversation short—and keeps effective treatment at bay.

In this book, I therefore pledge to present the best science available on girls with ADHD, to highlight optimal treatment strategies for such girls, and to present any wisdom I can on combating stigma—including the chance to see and hear some of the actual experiences that individuals and families encounter. (Please note: Unless explicitly identified, any case material in the pages that follow represents a composite of several individuals, with identities masked.) Overall, I aim to speak from both the heart and the science.

In the end, I will ask you to make some clear changes on your part, as parents, to understand the realities of ADHD, to stop blaming yourselves, and to pledge that you will deliver both unflagging warmth toward and clear limits on your daughter. This combination is not easy to implement, but doing any less will be a disservice. If we are to provide understanding, evidence-based clinical services, and stigma reduction regarding girls with ADHD, it will take honesty, resolve, love, and commitment.

Fasten your seat belts. There's a long and important road ahead. Welcome to the chapters that follow. The journey on which you're embarking could be life-changing for you, for your daughter, and for your entire family.

Acknowledgments

First, great thanks to the many participants, and their families, both those with ADHD and our neurotypical comparison girls and boys, who have been part of our team's summer program and treatment studies. Their allowing us to follow up with them over time has created much of the material in the pages of this book. Second, without the support of the National Institute of Mental Health, the U.S. Department of Education, and the National Institute on Drug Abuse, we could not have performed such research. Third, to my colleagues, students, and research assistants—too numerous to mention by name—I couldn't have done it without you! Fourth, Kitty Moore and Chris Benton of The Guilford Press have provided essential guidance and support throughout the entire process of creating this book. Fifth, I appreciate the helpful comments of Ashley Halkett and Dr. Kelly Campbell on drafts of many of the book's chapters. Finally, the love and support from (the same!) Kelly Campbell and our three sons, Jeff Hinshaw, John Neukomm, and Evan Hinshaw, have been instrumental.

ONE

What Does ADHD Look Like in Girls?

Let's start with a basic question that comes up all the time: Is ADHD—the acronym for *attention-deficit/hyperactivity disorder*—truly experienced by girls? I'm tempted to make this a much shorter chapter by limiting my answer to a single word: YES!

But as you might expect, there's a lot more to discuss.

Plus, you might need some convincing if you've heard the myth that ADHD does not occur in girls or women.

Many of you may be beginning to worry, regarding your daughter, about some of the issues and problems listed below:

- Messiness and disorganization
- Her seeming to be "out of it" for overly long periods of time
- Lack of forethought, then facing consequences after the fact, the hard way
- Excessive forgetfulness
- The appearance of not listening
- Getting unmotivated when the material to learn gets really tedious or hard
- Lack of restraint—"I have to do it *now!*"
- Defiance
- Overemotional nature
- Overtalking or excessive fidgeting
- Way too many "grudge matches" at home

- Generally poor self-control

- Just can't seem to get or stay organized

If this is the case, you may well be wondering: Is she just not trying? Or is she attempting to wear you down and get her own way for reasons that you can't quite understand? Why are you spending so much time talking with her teacher(s), or your friends and neighbors, wondering what on earth might be wrong? You may feel, as do many parents in similar situations, that at times you can relate to your daughter—yet at other moments you can't quite quell the suspicion that her schoolwork and friendships, along with your family's daily interactions, are slowly going down the drain.

Or maybe not so slowly.

Overall, for parents who deal with ADHD in their offspring, there's often a great deal of frustration—paired with self-blame ("What did I do during her early years to have caused all this?" or "Why can't I just say the right thing to her, ever?!"). In fact, soon enough I'll be asking you to work extremely hard on altering your expectations for a daughter with ADHD, involving a *radical acceptance* of her differences from other girls (sometimes subtle, sometimes quite overt) paired with a *radical commitment* to changing the family climate, altering many of your parenting strategies, and working in conjunction with her teachers, other school personnel, clinicians, and supports in the community.

What do I mean by the term *radical* here? It's taken from the language of a treatment called *dialectical behavior therapy* (DBT), which is a form of psychotherapy for individuals with severe emotion dysregulation and, often, self-injurious behaviors. *Radical* acceptance in DBT means that the person fully accepts her (or his) current reality—of difficult life events, or of longstanding personality traits—while letting go of the bitterness surrounding them. Such acceptance of life difficulties (working not to let them act as a continued source of stress and agony) can paradoxically help individuals do what they can to problem-solve in productive ways (hence, *radical* commitment to enacting change strategies). Without such shifts, the road ahead will be long and full of unexpected curves, too often accompanied by high "doses" of anger and self-recrimination.

With radical acceptance and commitment, challenges will still clearly await you, but thriving becomes a distinct possibility. I discuss these concepts later on in the book as well.

Does ADHD Really Occur in Girls?

What's the truth about ADHD? I'll be the first to admit: Things can be really hard to sort out in light of the torrent of conflicting information about ADHD circulating in the traditional media and social media, where polar-opposite views abound:

- ADHD is a myth—a made-up condition allowing pharmaceutical companies to promote the drugging of innocent children.

- ADHD is a biological label for kids who are exposed to lax parenting and unresponsive schools. If we just changed the way society is run, ADHD would not exist.

- ADHD emerges exclusively from the genes one was born with—and medications are the only valid treatment. In other words, parenting and schooling don't really matter because a girl's underlying genetics and biology are all that count.

- Forget Western medicine—herbal and alternative treatments are the only way to go for girls with what people consider to be the medical diagnosis of ADHD.

- Girls don't "have" ADHD—it's other conditions and diagnoses that are at play when a girl is showing poor self-control.

- ADHD should be diagnosed in girls just as much as in boys, after decades of professional neglect of female manifestations of the condition.

And this is only a tiny sample. A real challenge is how to sort myth from reality based on the extreme statements and viewpoints that seem to come out of the woodwork.

In fact, along with a large number of scientists and clinicians, I firmly believe that ADHD is a reality, although a complex one. It encompasses a range of genetic, biological, family- and school-related, and cultural forces that come together to yield real impairments in perhaps 4% of girls, worldwide. In fact, the diagnosis is a real possibility if the girl in question has longstanding and troublesome issues with self-regulation, good judgment, and self-motivation, particularly when these issues negatively affect her performance at home, at school, and with peers—or, at least, would do so without an incredible amount of outside support that might be keeping her barely afloat. At the same time, ADHD is not a diagnosis to be granted or received lightly. A host of other conditions can look a lot like it—and some may well accompany ADHD in a particular girl. Families need to take real care to obtain the best diagnostic work-up possible, as described in Chapter 2.

Still, when ADHD does exist in girls, the consequences can be monumental across a variety of important life areas, unless responsive support and intervention are put into action. The stakes are high.

> ADHD is real— and complex.

This chapter will help you start to build an understanding of whether your daughter might have ADHD and what you should do about it if she does (and even if she doesn't). It's frustrating for all of us that longstanding misconceptions—to the effect that ADHD is only a "male" condition—have led to a real shortage of information on girls with ADHD until quite recently. If ADHD does exist in girls, how often does it occur compared to in boys? Do the symptoms look the same or quite different? For far too long, many in the research, clinical, and educational fields have believed that ADHD is utterly rare, if not absent, in girls. At the same time, misunderstandings abound as to the different ways that ADHD can present itself in girls' cognitive abilities, behaviors, and emotions.

Rather than gently trickling from a lawn sprinkler, information about ADHD gushes from a fire hose these days. As such, it could take an entire book (actually, an entire series of books) to sort fact from fiction, reality from myth. At the end of this book I provide a Resources appendix that includes recommended materials for further reading and further action. For now, I attempt to present as clear and cogent an overview as I can, to put into context the experience and reality of youth, particularly girls, experiencing ADHD.

To begin with, let's pause to ask how we, as a society, consider children who have a *really* hard time with the demands of schooling. That is, children who don't seem to adapt well to requests to sit for long periods of time or acquire skills for which the human mind clearly wasn't evolved to attain, such as learning to read or do formal math. Expectations for acquiring these difficult cognitive skills have been present for only the past several thousand years of our species. In other words, we've been asking young children to do things that were never required in the 100,000-plus years of humankind before now. If you have an inborn difficulty with such functions, little wonder—in our achievement-oriented world these days—that there would be conflict, strife, and developmental problems.

I'm referring to kids whose parents bemoan them as "challenges," showing problems that surpass those of their siblings or other youth in the neighborhood or school, in terms of both frequency and intensity. Included are children and adolescents who seem to be slow to mature, which is particularly noticeable as societies demand, at ever-earlier ages, high levels of focus, achievement orientation, and the ability to go for long periods of time without significant rewards. Pressures to succeed academically and vocationally have never been stronger, so woe to the child who appears not to fit the mold—especially girls, whom most of us perceive as "naturally" more obedient and school-focused than boys.

Finally, an important note: Much of the material in this book is written as though there's a firm line between male/female or boy/girl. But as we are all increasingly realizing, it's not necessarily a binary division. In fact, as emphasized in an important post by Holly Miles and Christelle Thibault for the organization Inclusive Therapists—*www.inclusivetherapists.com/blog/the-intersection-of-adhd-and-gender-diversity*—all too little is known about the presence and experience of ADHD or other neurodevelopmental disorders in youth (or adults) who are "two-spirit, transgender, non-binary, gender-fluid, genderqueer, or agender." In fact, this is an area in great need of research. Overall, as you read further please realize that we all need to learn a lot more about ADHD in relation to gender diversity.

In short, as our expectations of how children need to develop have evolved, so have our views of problems like ADHD—which can erect obstacles to meeting those expectations. But the stereotypes of such youth pertain almost exclusively to boys. Let's explore this exclusion in some detail.

A Brief History of ADHD: Where Are the Girls?

Before the invention of the alphabet and written language, children with strong tendencies toward inattention, impulsivity, or hyperactivity may not have been recognized unless their problems were ultrasevere in the home or in the fields where they often worked alongside adults. Over the past several thousand years, only the children of royalty or the very wealthy were expected to learn to read and write. Yet even in preliterate, preagricultural societies, children displaying extreme problems with inattention or impulsive behavior might have been handicapped. Think of a preteen or teen in a hunter-gatherer society.

Some amount of risk taking and exploration may have led to discovery of the tribe's next meal. But an overly careless, rushed, and thoughtless style, involving a lack of attention and planning on the "hunt," may have led to misfires with a rock, spear, or bow and arrow, leaving the tribe desperately hungry.

Still, it's no coincidence that depictions of what is now termed ADHD began to emerge in the medical and educational communities when compulsory education became prevalent, in the early 1800s and beyond. Any child whose negative behavior (in a mandatory classroom) was disruptive might well threaten the learning of all classmates. (Think of the one-room schoolhouses in rural areas, or more factory-like classrooms in urban districts, where behavioral control was at a premium.) Extremes of distractibility, poor impulse control, and the inability to sit still for long periods at a time would stand out like a sore thumb.

But girls unable to meet these expectations have been a perpetual mystery. Boys were typically expected to be mischievous and unruly, but a girl showing these tendencies was believed to be far outside the norm. Even more, girls with difficulties in self-regulation were (and still are) less likely than boys to show truly disruptive, obstreperous, or oppositional behavior. Instead, their more frequent problems with inattention, disorganization, and careless mistakes were (and still are) not as bothersome to adults.

> Girls with the hallmark symptoms of ADHD are still often thought to have some other problem.

To this day, teachers may actually be relieved that such girls can at least follow basic classroom rules for deportment. Fortunately, the last three decades have seen recognition of ADHD in girls finally come of age. But even now, the core view in medicine, psychology, and education remains in place that girls with core issues in compliance, attention, and self-control must have something far different from ADHD at the root of their problems.

It Was All about (Mis)Behavior . . .

How did we get here? Let's look back at how ADHD was conceptualized early in its history. When compulsory schooling began to take hold, the medical profession struggled to account for children who had at least average intellectual abilities, experienced no vision or hearing loss, and were able to recognize reality (that is, not be overtly psychotic)—but nonetheless showed major difficulties with self-regulation, rule following, and the ability to sustain attention and resist distraction. Just after the turn of the 20th century, a notable account specifically described these kinds of children (noted to be predominantly boys) as having a "defect in moral control." This description did not mean that such children were inherently "immoral" but instead that they had major issues with regulating their behavior in accordance with social and adult norms. Unfortunately, the connotation of such children as "bad" or immoral has not entirely left our views, even today.

I believe that this is a particular burden for girls. During the first several years of life, girls mature earlier than boys in empathy, language capacity, and brain development. Therefore, it often seems completely unnatural (or even immoral) for a girl to lack self-control, have trouble with school materials, defy teachers, and/or act younger than her age. Because of the importance of social interactions for both girls and women, female peers are particularly apt to dislike and reject girls with the core signs of ADHD more frequently than boys dislike and reject fellow males with ADHD. In short, from both adults and other youth, a particular stigma surrounds girls with ADHD that outstrips such disapproval and denigration for boys.

> *Because we expect more self-control and social skill from girls, we often judge those who fall short due to ADHD more harshly than boys with ADHD.*

Then It Was a Disorder of the Brain . . .

Over time, professionals have emphasized different aspects of the underlying behavior patterns as the core symptoms, applying a variety of diagnoses and labels to such patterns. Labels for much of the 20th century focused on such terms as brain injury, brain damage, organic brain disease, or minimal brain dysfunction. Or the terms focused on deficits, as in *clumsy child syndrome*.

Interestingly though tragically, the influenza pandemic of 1918–1919 left millions dead but also survivors who emerged with distinctive problems in concentration, self-control, learning, and other behavioral features that closely resemble what we today call ADHD. As a result, diagnoses such as brain damage or brain injured became common for the next 50 years. The assumption was that any person who could not behave properly in school or work, and who showed erratic problems of self-regulation and focus, must have an underlying brain pathology. Certainly, as discussed in later chapters (see especially Chapter 4), many ADHD-style behaviors have biological as opposed to exclusively psychological origins. But these diagnoses were used indiscriminately to signal a huge range of problematic behaviors and emotional displays. Even more, because of the untested assumption that brain damage was always the cause, the labels discounted the roles of parents, teachers, schools, and communities at large in shaping an individual child's outcomes.

. . . and Then Back to Behavior

By the middle of the 20th century, there were two opposing trends. One was to soften earlier labels related to brain damage as minimal brain dysfunction, which (as just noted) incorporated many problems well beyond what we currently conceptualize as ADHD. Another was to focus more specifically on the actual motor behaviors of the condition: fidgeting, squirming, being unable to sit still, and the like. As a result, terms like *hyperkinesis*, *hyperkinetic impulse disorder*, and *hyperactivity* took hold. The problem with that approach was that girls don't display these problems to nearly the same extent as do boys, which contributed to insufficient recognition that girls could have this kind of problem. Inattentive symptoms got lost in the shuffle.

A Lag in Development

Intriguingly, a research-based trend emerged in the 1950s to brand the behavioral problems of inattentiveness, forgetfulness, poor impulse control, and overactivity as reflecting an "immaturity syndrome" in children. As it turns out (and is presented as a key point in Chapter 4), what is now termed *ADHD* does in fact denote behaviorally and emotionally immature children and teens. Yet this did not immediately help clinicians or the public recognize ADHD in girls.

The Emergence of ADD—and Then ADHD

Finally, in the 1970s and 1980s, Canadian psychologist Virginia Douglas proposed that the inability to "stop, look, and listen" was the core of the condition. In other words, at its foundation were difficulties in attending to the environment, restraining impulses, considering the actual contingencies of the situation (at home, in the classroom, in peer groups), and adapting one's behavior to the context at hand. The American Psychiatric Association therefore branded the condition as ADD (attention deficit disorder), which may or may not be accompanied by hyperactivity. Thus, the terms *ADD with hyperactivity* and *ADD without hyperactivity* were born. Not so many years later, the awkward term ADHD took hold, with the explicit suggestion that both attention deficits and hyperactivity could be present. Note that today many people, including health and mental health professionals, use the terms *ADHD* and *ADD* interchangeably. They are actually the same thing, although ADD can now often refer to the inattentive symptoms without the hyperactive/impulsive ones.

How Is ADHD Defined?

In the latest versions of the classification systems used in the United States and in other countries, ADHD is held to be composed of the following:

- Extremely high levels of inattentive/distractible/forgetful behaviors, typically leading to poor follow-through and poor rule-following at home and school
- Extremely high levels of acting before thinking about the consequences of the action, choosing the first response rather than considering a range of responses, interrupting others, excessively fidgeting, and having trouble containing the desire to keep moving
- Or both of the above

Children and youth with exclusive inattention/disorganization are branded as having the *inattentive presentation* of ADHD (ADHD–Inattentive), those with exclusive hyperactivity/impulsivity as exhibiting the *hyperactive/impulsive presentation* (ADHD–Hyperactive/Impulsive), and those with both symptom domains as having the *combined presentation* (ADHD–Combined). The hyperactive/impulsive form shows up mainly in preschoolers and overwhelmingly in boys. As highlighted throughout this book, girls are more likely than boys to display the inattentive form. Still, many girls with ADHD display considerable impulsivity as well as inattention and disorganization.

Official diagnostic guidelines specify that a girl (or a boy) must show a requisite number of symptoms of inattention and/or hyperactivity/impulsivity for at least half a year, with some of them appearing before age 12. Those symptoms must interfere with the child's development or with functioning in at least two domains of life, such as at home and at school—or in social interactions and at school.

If your daughter fits the picture of inattention, she may have a really hard time following directions. She may not remember what she's supposed to do at home or school, even when it would be ingrained in other kids because of the routine. She might seem to focus on almost anything other than what she's supposed to be focusing on (like homework, or what you're telling her about a weekend outing)—in other words, she seems extremely distractible. Commonly, she loses things and her surroundings are far from organized. Although she "gets" the content of many if not most of her school subjects, she typically gets worse grades than she should because of a lot of careless mistakes (in other words, she may see the forest but misses out on a lot of trees close by). Finishing tasks is a major headache, for her and you, as well as her teacher(s). Although she is typically highly engaged in activities she likes or at which she thrives, motivation seems to flag quickly when there are many steps to a chore or assignment—or the timeframe is relatively long for completing it. Girls with the inattentive form of ADHD often show many (or even all) of these patterns, but they aren't as active, dangerous, thoughtless, impulsive, or rude/bossy as those who score high on the hyperactive/impulsive group of issues.

So, what do these hyperactive/impulsive behaviors look like? If your daughter fits this pattern, you might be seeing, first, a lot of movement: squirming while seated, leaving the dinner table repeatedly, tapping feet/ hands or otherwise keeping in a kind of constant motion, or showing a real physical energy to climb or simply move fast. (*Note:* As highlighted later in the book, girls may be more prone than boys to be more hyperverbal than hyperactive per se.) In fact, impulsive behaviors include real difficulty waiting in line, frequent interrupting of others, answering in class (or on test questions) immediately—without giving full thought before responding, making lots of noise during supposedly quiet activities, and sometimes doing dangerous things for the fun or thrill of it.

It's rare for a child above the age of 5 or 6 to display high levels solely on this second list of hyperactive/impulsive symptoms. That is, once they are in grade school, the combined form of ADHD involves lots of inattentive *and* hyperactive/impulsive behaviors.

It is extremely important not to diagnose children and teens simply because they display high levels of these problems: They also need to be experiencing considerable life problems as a result. These impairments at home and school are probably what brought you to this book, and any clinician you see should consider diagnosing your daughter with ADHD only when the problems yield real mismatches with the behavioral standards of home life, classrooms, or relationships with peers. Furthermore, the symptoms should not be attributable to other serious conditions (such as depression), even though such conditions may well exist alongside ADHD.

> *Impairment should be considered more important to diagnosis than the number of ADHD symptoms.*

Problems with the Diagnostic Criteria—Especially for Girls

You can probably tell at this point that diagnosing ADHD is no simple matter. That's why you need a well-qualified clinician to evaluate your daughter (as described in Chapter 2). But be aware that there are a few glitches in the current diagnostic criteria:

- *The requirement that symptoms must appear before age 12 can really penalize girls—because for many girls with really impairing ADHD these issues don't emerge fully until middle school and beyond.*

- *Calling this a disorder of attention is incomplete and misleading.* The key problem for those with ADHD is not poor attention per se but a fundamental difficulty in *regulating attention as the demands of a given task, project, or situation shift.*

For example, ever heard of *hyperfocus?* This is a state in which one has real trouble coming back to earth when deeply engaged in a set of thoughts, a highly motivating project, or a video game, often for hours at a time. Many individuals with ADHD, *especially girls and women,* can focus quite well—or even hyperfocus—on tasks or activities in which they are inherently interested. But for rote or boring tasks, or those requiring extensive planning and organization, their interest, attention, and engagement quickly fizzle out. So, ADHD isn't a simple problem of not being able to focus or pay attention. Instead, it's a higher-order issue reflecting the ability to *regulate* or modulate one's effort, focus, and attention (hence the terms *poor self-control* or *poor self-regulation*).

● *Assessments focusing on any specific individual tests may miss the mark because individuals with ADHD tend to be "consistently inconsistent" across a wide range of tests.* Scientists have been using all sorts of cognitive tests and tasks in research studies to help pin down the problem. (Aha! ADHD is a deficit in "selective attention" or "sustained attention" or "the ability to resist distraction," and so on.) But summing across these studies reveals that those with ADHD are not inevitably worse on any particular cognitive or attentional task. Instead, their performance is highly variable and erratic over repeated trials on many different tests and measures. In short, people with ADHD have major issues with lapses in motivation and attention, which means their performance can easily vary from situation to situation or time to time. So, it's not one particular kind of task on which their highly variable performance is an issue; it's on several. People with ADHD waver between attention and distraction, focus and noninterest, on-task behavior and lapses in performance. If your daughter truly has ADHD, her underlying performance is likely to be erratic, for reasons that are not under her (or your) immediate control.

● *Almost all of the information gathered on ADHD is based on studies of boys.* Hovering over all of this is the fact that just about all of the information on ADHD, and what constitutes its essence, comes from thousands of studies that involve either all boys or extremely high ratios of boys to girls. As a result, we are not positive whether the trove of information on ADHD from the history of research on the topic truly applies to females. This goes not only for the kinds of problems they display but also for underlying issues such as brain mechanisms and other forces that may drive their chances for positive or negative outcomes. My own research team, in parallel with others, has pioneered intensive studies of the behavior patterns, life problems, underlying causes, treatment responses, and long-term outcomes of girls with ADHD. Throughout this book, I attempt to intersperse our wisdom and our findings into the information provided.

In the end, understanding female ADHD is essential if our knowledge base is to grow, so that information for you as parents—and for educators, clinicians, and the general public—isn't based on exclusively male-related facts and theories. Only by understanding ADHD in girls and women can health care professionals begin to assess and treat it accurately in females.

How Prevalent Is ADHD in Girls Compared to Boys?

This is not as easy a question to answer as you might think. The answer depends on how ADHD is measured and defined (and the contexts in which it exists), what kinds of samples are studied (those coming to clinics or those in the general population), and the kinds of ADHD symptoms in question. See the box on pages 14–15 for details. We still have not perfected how we study the incidence of ADHD, and how the rate in girls precisely compares to that in boys, but we are making headway.

Even so, I believe that during childhood more boys than girls do have ADHD. Most surveys done throughout the 20th century—especially when the surveys were of youth in treatment of some kind—revealed 5:1, 10:1, or even far higher boy:girl ratios. Not only were the samples biased (for example, boys have higher rates of associated aggressive behaviors than girls, and it's typically such behaviors that get a child referred for assessment and treatment), but there was little or no differentiation of inattention from hyperactivity/impulsivity in rating scales until 1980, when the concept of ADD took hold.

The research deck is stacked toward identifying boys with ADHD.

Things have changed in recent years. Symptom lists are now divided into inattentive versus hyperactivity/impulsivity items, and population-based surveys have become government priorities and are performed more regularly. Also, awareness has risen in health professionals and the general public alike that ADHD in girls is a reality.

Accordingly, national surveys of random households with respect to ADHD show a smaller, but still male-dominated, boy:girl ratio of between 2:1 and 2.5:1. The National Survey of Children's Health (NSCH), a random sample of 100,000 families contacted by phone and repeated every few years, is one significant example. In 2003, for the first time, ADHD-specific questions were included in the survey, inquiring about children in the household between 4 and 17 years of age. Specifically, the parent was asked whether the child had a current diagnosis of ADD or ADHD. The question was then repeated about whether the child had *ever* received such a diagnosis. Of course, we cannot know if the diagnosis was made accurately, but it reflects current professional

Why the Difference in the Rate of ADHD between Girls and Boys Is Difficult to Measure Accurately

Here are some of the reasons that the differences in prevalence between boys and girls are hard to measure with complete accuracy.

- Measures and cutoff points are floating targets. (1) We have few objective measures of brain or bodily processes linked with ADHD to add to reports of observations by parents and teachers. (2) We're also looking at a condition that is not in a "yes or no" illness category (like cancer) but instead represents extreme scores along a continuum—of inattention and/or hyperactivity/impulsivity for ADHD. (3) The precise number of symptoms used to determine the presence of ADHD is an educated guess. Interestingly, good evidence exists that when observing objectively similar levels of ADHD behaviors in boys and girls, adults attribute those problems to ADHD far more for boys than they do for girls. In other words, the very rating-scale measures used to assess ADHD may be biased.

- Let's take the example of two 9-year-old girls. Amanda has the requisite number of ADHD symptoms, but does not exhibit significant impairment, because of her strong cognitive abilities, along with good family and classroom supports. She can't therefore qualify for a diagnosis. Lizzy, with the exact same symptom counts, is seriously compromised academically by problems in learning, her overly rigid school setting, and her lack of structure at home regarding homework expectations. She therefore receives a clear diagnosis. The point here is that with respect to ADHD—along with just about all other mental health, learning, and neurodevelopmental conditions—the symptom counts exist in contexts (home, school, community), as well as cultures, all of which play a huge role in shaping the way the symptoms are displayed and appraised. The same contexts can either exacerbate impairments or foster resilient functioning.

- Research samples don't accurately represent the general population. For practical purposes, many studies use children in clinical settings, who tend to be the ones with the worst problems, or those with families who can afford services, or those who differ in other important ways from the rest of the children who would meet diagnostic criteria. They don't really represent the general population. It has taken a long time in the United States for estimates of ADHD in boys versus girls to benefit from studies of non-clinically-referred children, truly representing the population.

- Until recent years, the two symptom domains have not been separated out in research. Because girls in the general population display considerably lower rates of hyperactive/impulsive behaviors than boys, but with relatively equivalent rates of inattention, failing to separate the two domains means not truly representing girls.

practices. If the answers were "yes," the follow-up question was whether the child or adolescent had ever received medication for ADD or ADHD. Some interesting findings from the NSCH are in the box on page 16.

Is This a True Sex Difference?

In short, current information confirms that ADHD occurs more often in boys than in girls, although the difference is not as great as once thought. Without reliable biological measures, however, we still can't be sure that these findings aren't related to an ongoing bias toward identifying males. I believe nonetheless that the numbers are reasonably accurate. Here's why:

- *A higher rate of ADHD among boys is consistent with the higher rates of other neurodevelopmental disorders among boys.* Neurodevelopmental disorders, like ADHD, typically start early in life and involve core issues in cognitive, social, and behavioral deviations and delays. Other neurodevelopmental conditions include autism spectrum disorders, Tourette syndrome, many learning disorders, and—in the views of some—early conduct disturbances that involve frank defiance and aggressive behavior from a very early age. Taking a broad view of many relevant studies, boys display higher rates of all such neurodevelopmental disorders. Overall, the first 10 years of life constitute the risk period for boys with respect to the onset of neurodevelopmental conditions, including ADHD.

- *Girls exhibit faster brain development in early life than boys do, and boys have higher rates of conditions that reflect their slower development.* As noted earlier, over the first few years of life, girls show higher levels of behavioral control, empathy, impulse control, compliance, and language development than boys. So, it stands to reason that conditions involving social awareness and

What We Have Learned about ADHD in Girls
from the NSCH

- Between 2003 and 2012, the percentage of all children ages 4–17 who had ever been diagnosed with ADHD, per parent report, climbed 41%!

- Specifically, by 2012, 11% of all children had received a diagnosis—which is one in nine (and well above rates in just about every other country on earth).

- The boy:girl ratio was about 2.3:1.

- By 2012, and now replicated in other large surveys, lower-income youth slightly outnumbered middle- or upper-class youth and Black children and adolescents slightly outnumbered White children and adolescents. Things have changed since the early days of the "Tom Sawyer" syndrome of the ADHD diagnosis being reserved almost exclusively for White, relatively affluent boys.

- By the time of the 2016 survey, the age range of the children had been extended to 2–17 years. Of course, very few 2- to 3-year-olds get diagnosed with ADHD. The numbers stayed at or just above the 2012 levels. The boy:girl ratio remained at about 2.3:1.

- *For the time being, girls are receiving diagnoses far more than they did a generation or two ago.*

- Finally, what's also intriguing about the NSCH data is that in the rising rates of ADHD diagnoses, for both boys and girls, there is a massive state-by-state variation. In some states (mainly in the South and Midwest), rates are two to three times higher than in the far West. There could be many factors involved here, but at least one pertains to whether states prioritize public-school test scores at all costs. It is just those states that witness the largest increases in rates of ADHD diagnoses, especially for the poorest youth in the state. Policies emphasizing academic performance at all costs may help to increase the pressure to diagnose ADHD.

language development (autism), self-regulation (ADHD, early conduct disturbance), and motor control (Tourette) show higher rates in boys than in girls. In all, the first decade of life is the risk period for boy-dominated neurodevelopmental conditions.

An important note: During the second 10 years of life, girls skyrocket ahead of boys with respect to emotional (sometimes called "internalizing") disorders like depression, serious anxiety, eating problems, and self-harm. This is a big story, which I discuss in more detail later in the book. Yet it is of real relevance to girls with underlying ADHD, as their risk for such internalizing problems is markedly enhanced during the crucial teen years, over and above rates for other adolescent females.

Finally, and intriguingly, the sex ratio with respect to ADHD becomes much closer to even by adulthood. In other words, just about as many women as men qualify for an ADHD diagnosis. This is a fascinating puzzle, which I consider in later chapters.

Why Were Girls Overlooked Regarding ADHD for So Long?

I learned as a graduate student back in the 1970s and 1980s that ADHD was basically a male-only condition. This was the professional and scientific standard. Indeed, the very rating scales used by parents and teachers to detect behavioral and emotional problems in children were typically loaded with "ADHD" items emphasizing overt hyperactivity and behavioral impulsivity rather than inattention per se. As I've already noted, girls are more likely than boys to have the exclusively inattentive type of ADHD, and these scales did not adequately represent relevant symptoms in girls. These inattentive-type symptoms are also rather "quiet" in classrooms, meaning that they're less disruptive and noticeable to teachers. When they are noticed, they are often believed to emanate from depression or anxiety.

But there is more to the story than this.

The problem of major male overrepresentation in research and clinical recognition goes far beyond ADHD. In fact, even basic animal research on physiology and behavior is biased toward males in a whole range of species. In humans, medical studies of cardiovascular disease, and resultant heart attacks, were so focused on men that there simply wasn't enough information to understand the potentially different risk factors and interventions that relate to women.

In the early 1990s, the U.S. National Institutes of Health began to require that all research studies funded by the various institutes—ranging from cancer to pulmonary disease, from infectious illness to mental disorders—include females to the greatest extent possible. Parallel guidelines then emerged for inclusion of children and adolescents, as well as socioeconomically and racially diverse samples. Without full representation, our scientific models and clinical practices will simply be off-base. Yet progress has been slower than hoped. Established biases, plus long-held beliefs that male sex is the sole standard, are hard to break.

Girls have truly suffered in silence for far too many years. We still have a long way to go, but things are finally changing.

What Does ADHD in Girls Actually Look Like?

A number of girls with ADHD qualify for the combined form of the condition, meaning that they show lots of inattentive *and* hyperactive/impulsive symptoms. These are the girls most likely to display oppositionality and defiance, with problems not only in school but also with their peers (who may be bewildered by their intrusive, bossy, and seemingly insensitive style) and with authority figures. My team and I have worked with a large number of girls with ADHD over the years, and many mirror the kinds of defiant, ornery, "my-way-or-the-highway" stances of boys. But even here, subtle but important differences are apparent:

• Hyperactivity in girls is much more likely to appear as mental restlessness than the types of physical restlessness that boys experience. Your daughter might feel like she can't slow her thoughts down or get them into some linear configuration.

• Instead of the overly active movements of boys, girls with combined-type ADHD are prone to exhibit overly intense verbal behavior. Your daughter might constantly interrupt others or seem to believe that her views are the only ones worth stating. These symptoms should be emphasized in the assessment of girls and women, over and above physical manifestations of impulsivity and overactivity per se, which are the hallmarks in boys.

Yet even more, as noted earlier, girls are simply more likely than boys to present with the inattentive symptoms of ADHD as the main or even exclusive feature. These, as it turns out, are important factors in the long-term outcome for girls with ADHD.

> Even when girls have the "same" ADHD symptoms as boys, the manifestation of those symptoms can be very different.

What Happens When Girls with ADHD Grow Older?

It's important to note, first, that until relatively recently, we simply haven't known about the long-term outcomes of girls with ADHD, because of the lack of recognition of girls with this condition—which greatly curtailed any research at all with females, and particularly any research beyond childhood. However, a number of small investigations, and two much larger ones, have finally provided some guidance with respect to expectations for outcome:

- On average, girls with carefully diagnosed ADHD continue to struggle with academic performance as well as many cognitive functions, relationships with peers and adults, self-concept, and need for additional services. They are also prone to experiencing additional psychological, behavioral, and emotional problems into adolescence and adulthood.

- Evidence is conflicting as to whether girls with ADHD, as they grow older, have higher rates of substance abuse and eating disorders than their typically developing peers. Some girls, however, clearly show such risk.

- Strong evidence is now emerging that girls with ADHD, by adolescence and early adulthood, show a marked tendency toward engaging in self-harm, including frank suicidal behavior. Rates of unplanned pregnancy and poor performance on the job are also strikingly high.

The hyperactive/impulsive symptoms that dominate in boys during childhood may receive a lot of (negative) attention from parents and teachers. These can predict later problems for girls who display high levels as well, especially related to later involvement in aggression and engagement in forms of self-harm like cutting and self-mutilation. Yet it's actually the high levels and high intensity of inattentive problems that predict a range of difficult adult outcomes. Inattentiveness—more precisely, as I've discussed, the lack of ability to regulate attention—is heavily involved in later academic problems, issues with driving, engagement in substance abuse, on-the-job performance, and other difficult issues in adolescence and beyond, including self-harm. Unless we pay careful attention to the attention-related and organization-related problems so characteristic of girls with ADHD, we will miss the boat.

Let's take an example. A young woman with ADHD has been working hard for six months at her job, but realizes that she now has a new shift supervisor. This supervisor soon comments that the young woman is falling behind on daily reports that need to be made—related to her underlying inattention and disorganization. After the supervisor's critical comment (though it was intended to be helpful), the employee fires off a nasty e-mail reply and texts coworkers, calling out the supervisor's insensitivity. Here, the long-standing attentional problems—accompanied by an overly impulsive, hasty, and defensive retort—have sparked a fast-growing work crisis. Note that the impulsive response may not have been as overtly hostile as one that a male employee might have made, but even the indirect and more subtle lack of restraint escalated the situation.

Furthermore, girls often engage in a lot more behaviors intended to compensate for ADHD symptoms than boys do. You may see your daughter overstudying, refusing to give up, holding to perfectionistic standards, or working day and night. If these habits help her perform well, they might obscure the fact that she has ADHD, at least until the bar is raised in middle school, high school, or college. And what about the costs of such superhuman efforts? Your daughter may end up sacrificing sleep, exercise, mindful eating, and recreation, with accumulated stress bound to take a toll. Also, it's the period between childhood and adolescence when serious issues of anxiety, depression, and even self-harm are likely to emerge for all girls. When ADHD is already present, the risk is even higher.

In all, the factors that make ADHD hard to detect in preteen girls may actually spur difficult and even self-punitive behavior patterns as they mature.

At the same time, however, such major problems are not inevitable. We continue to search for the processes that can drive positive and resilient outcomes. So I close this section with an essential takeaway message. Namely, girls (and women) who get diagnosed with ADHD are *not* all the same. Not only are symptom profiles different, especially between girls with exclusive inattention as opposed to the combined form—but girls bring different temperaments, personality styles, coping mechanisms, family support, and classroom skills to the table. It's a hugely mistaken assumption to categorize all girls with ADHD (as well as all boys with ADHD) as more similar to one another than different from one another. Finding each girl's individual strengths as well as weaknesses, along with the specific actions and activities that "make her tick" or trigger her, are crucial to healthy outcomes. This is an important task for you as her parent and her advocate—even though finding bright spots can seem quite challenging when the family seems entangled in the problems linked to her ADHD. I return to all of these issues later in this book.

So What Do You Do If Your Daughter Has ADHD?

This is the core question for the rest of the book. What can you do to help? To start out, be sure that your daughter gets the kind of evidence-based evaluation outlined in Chapter 2 and that it reveals that she does indeed fit the profile for an ADHD diagnosis. Even though ADHD is not a fixed "box" within which all girls are the same, it probably does mean that your daughter shares a number of characteristics with other girls or teens who fall under this classification.

So you're now on a journey. It will be a long journey, and one for which the outcome can't yet be predicted. But at its outset, here are some issues to confront.

First, you'll need to adapt and change your perspective on your daughter, yourself, and your family. You might initially feel disbelief or denial: *This isn't who my daughter is! She's more than just a diagnostic label.* You might feel anger: *How dare the psychological or medical profession claim that she's just like all those other girls I read about in the press or on social media!?* Alternatively, it might dawn on you that everything you've kept at bay for so long—the suspicion that a longstanding pattern underlying her erratic, underfocused, and troublesome behavior—might actually have an explanation, which could now bring some solace and point to a road toward getting help.

Please remember the concepts of *radical acceptance* and *radical commitment* introduced at the beginning of this chapter. You will need to accept that your daughter is not entirely like many of her peers—and that it will take a lot of work to give her the coping skills that she needs.

Even more, if you're her biological parent, you might come to recognize that her relatives, at least some of them, share similar characteristics. Maybe even you! As I discuss in later chapters, ADHD is transmitted more through shared genes than through environmental factors. If it turns out that you have ADHD, you may inadvertently exacerbate such patterns in your daughter through your own lack of organization and planning, your own issues with anger management, or your own restless and impulsive style. Or through simple frustration over your daughter's differences.

Speaking of parenting styles, it's a mistake to think that negative parenting is the true cause of ADHD (the genetic predisposition is real, as is emphasized in Chapter 4). But it's also incorrect to think that, because genes have a lot to say about an individual's likelihood of developing ADHD, parenting doesn't matter at all. This is an all-too-common misconception. In fact, even for conditions shaped exclusively by inherited genes, how those genetic predispositions are either fueled or reduced by environments can make all the difference for later thriving.

In other words, for ADHD, where genetics and biology play an indisputable role, parents cannot afford to take on the blame for their child's lapses. Doing so is demoralizing and simply inaccurate. Yet at the same time, it's essential for parents and families (whether biological or adoptive) to take the responsibility to examine their own parenting styles, strive for greater consistency, obtain the best possible support for themselves, and participate in interventions aimed at helping their child's learning and behavioral issues.

More simply: Stop the self-blame, but take responsibility.

At another level, as noted above, you may clearly benefit from trying for a kind of radical acceptance of your daughter's differences. Some of these differences may drive you mad, a lot of the time or even most of the time. But if she finds the right kinds of parental acceptance, nurturance, and support; the right kinds of educational guidance; and the right kinds of strength promotion—she may well gain competence and confidence, with the potential to make uncommon contributions in her life and touch the lives of many others.

The take-home message is this: I don't subscribe to the view that ADHD is an inevitable, hidden gift. In fact, the negative consequences are all too common and, by now, well documented. But I do believe that the kinds of out-of-the-box thinking, intense drive, and ability to go beyond common perspectives and solutions can propel girls with ADHD to make a real mark on the world.

> *Don't put yourself down, but do take hold of the reins.*

Remember to get as much support as you can from families who've already been down this road. Engaging in treatments that have stood the test of time is crucial. We in the scientific community certainly still need to develop, test, and disseminate newer and more effective interventions. But try not to become overly enamored of the "best new thing" you find on the internet, as many such postings are entirely devoid of any scientific basis.

Remember, ADHD doesn't just vanish as your daughter goes through adolescence and makes the gradual transition to adulthood. In fact, it can actually intensify, in both expected and unexpected ways. Best to head things off at the pass, to the greatest extent possible, with treatments that show the best evidence of success. Much more regarding treatments follows later in the book.

Is ADHD All There Is?

This is one of the most crucial questions that you can ask. It's one that directly confronts both those who scientifically investigate and clinically treat girls with ADHD and, of course, all parents dealing with ADHD in their offspring.

A huge amount of research reveals that most girls (and boys) with core problems of inattention and hyperactivity/impulsivity typically have one or more—and sometimes many more—problems that accompany ADHD. More detail on these so-called *comorbidities* can be found in Chapter 2, but here's an overview:

● *Anxiety*. First, there can be significant anxiety, defined as the experience of worry, dread, or even terror without a true threat present. Excessive worrying, a feeling of constant tension, avoidance of situations that seem to trigger the anxiety, fast breathing or rapid heartbeat, and unexplained pain are some key signs of the various anxiety disorders one might experience. Sometimes the sheer stress of having ADHD may trigger anxiety reactions, particularly around school and schoolwork. In other cases, serious anxiety conditions predate ADHD. One of the points of potential confusion here is that a feeling of restlessness can be a sign of anxiety—but restlessness is also a symptom of ADHD. Finally, one of the more difficult issues for a clinician is to make the distinction, particularly for girls, between the inattentive presentation of ADHD and a true anxiety disorder. This kind of "differential diagnosis" (that is, figuring out what belongs where) can be tricky because many girls with inattentive-style ADHD are not at all hyperactive; instead, they are often rather quiet, inhibited, and highly anxious about school and home issues. All this is important because anxiety disorders require different treatment strategies than ADHD itself does.

● *Depression*. Beyond the sadness we all encounter as part of the human condition, major depression involves at least two weeks of out-of-the-ordinary sadness and dark mood (or in some cases a kind of blankness or absence of mood), loss of motivation, repetitive thoughts of self-criticism, sleep and appetite disturbance, and social withdrawal. At its extremes, depression can prompt the belief that life isn't worth living. One of the symptoms of depression is poor concentration, often related to the negative, ruminative thoughts and utterly low motivation the girl is experiencing. So, the clinician will need to tease out what's depression and what's ADHD. Although some preteen girls with ADHD experience depression, the number grows greatly by adolescence, the time period during which depression takes hold in a large number of adolescent girls. Like anxiety, depression requires different forms of treatment than ADHD, so it's really important to know whether it is an accompaniment.

• *Bipolar disorder.* This is a serious condition in which depressive episodes either alternate with or occur simultaneously with periods of mania, marked by sped-up thinking and behavior, serious impulsivity, fast-shifting moods (during which feelings of elation or superiority can emerge), irritability, and increased motivation for pleasurable events (even if dangerous). The careful reader will notice that impulsivity and irritability can also be a core part of ADHD, so differential diagnosis is especially important here. Bipolar disorder can begin during childhood, but the highest risk period is in mid to late adolescence and beyond. Professionals now know that bipolar disorder can coexist with ADHD. In fact, with a high family "loading" of mood disorders, a history of ADHD in childhood can emerge as bipolar disorder by the teen or early adult years. Medication treatment for bipolar disorder typically involves different primary medications than medications for ADHD, though sometimes the two types of medication can be combined.

• *Oppositional behavior and conduct problems.* Many boys with ADHD—especially those with the combined form, which includes impulsivity and hyperactivity—are hard to manage, defiant with respect to adult requests, and oppositional seemingly whenever limits are set. For a subgroup, such early oppositional defiant disorder can develop into conduct disorder, a far more serious condition involving severe rule-breaking, fighting and other forms of aggression, running away from home, and the like. Girls with ADHD can certainly experience these conditions as well, particularly those with the combined form. More than boys, however, such girls often engage in relational aggression. That is, instead of physically confronting their peers, they may attempt to ruin reputations through the spreading of rumors or "backstabbing" via other means. Think of the potential for such actions to do harm with the fast rise of social media in the past few years. Fortunately, family- and school-based treatments for oppositional defiant disorder and conduct disorder are similar to those that are effective for ADHD.

• *Learning disorders.* Girls with ADHD often struggle with schoolwork related to their inattentive/disorganized symptoms. Yet learning disorders—in reading, math, or writing—have more to do with below-age-expected deficiencies in the underlying language, visual, cognitive, and motor problems related to literacy or numerical operations. Many girls with such learning disorders are inattentive when they try to learn or practice these skills—because such tasks are inherently difficult for them—but are otherwise relatively self-regulated. As noted above, girls with ADHD show poor attention regulation with regard to a wide variety of requests, beyond school subjects per se. Again, a careful differential diagnosis is essential. Still, a quarter or more of girls with ADHD also experience specific learning disorders. For them, specialized academic programs are needed, beyond evidence-based treatments for ADHD.

 • *Posttraumatic stress disorder (PTSD).* I'll take up this topic at more length in Chapter 4, but the key point for now is that when girls have experienced early trauma—not just natural disasters but also including exposure to family or neighborhood violence, physical abuse, or sexual abuse—inattentive and sometimes impulsive problems can emerge. In fact, some critics of an overly biological perspective contend that ADHD is the result of trauma more than of genetic inheritance—and that it would be a great mistake to give medications to such girls on the basis of a careless diagnosis of ADHD. Yet consider the following: (1) ADHD and PTSD can actually overlap, rather than serving as totally distinct entities; and (2) trauma in children can produce physical and brain-related responses. It's not *either–or*; it could be *both–and*. Once more, only a careful diagnostic work-up can distinguish relevant personal histories or make the determination that ADHD and PTSD coexist.

Finally, when adolescence hits, as I've already noted, the teen years can bring on depression or bipolar disorder, more so than in childhood. Other conditions that can emerge in adolescence (if not before), particularly for girls with ADHD, are substance use conditions, eating disorders, and self-harm. I'll save detailed discussion of these until Chapter 9, when we take up adolescent issues for girls with ADHD in much more detail.

Overall, ADHD may well *not* be all that's going on. In the next chapter, therefore, I cover essentials of assessment and evaluation related not only to ADHD but also to such additional areas of concern. I will delve more deeply into what the conditions described in broad strokes here may look like to you and to your daughter's teachers—and how a qualified professional will evaluate your child to ensure that your daughter gets the best help possible. That's always the goal of diagnosis—figuring out how to provide the best possible life for your child.

TWO

Does Your Daughter
Have ADHD?

Now that you know what ADHD looks like in girls, my aim in this chapter is to walk you through the assessment and evaluation procedures that can give you the best idea of whether your daughter has ADHD. We'll go inside the evaluator's office to see what kinds of measures, interviews, and tests are most useful.

But in order to obtain the information that's needed, assessments must go far beyond the clinician's office. As you undoubtedly sense already, ADHD reveals itself at mealtimes, during homework sessions, in interactions with friends, and particularly at school. It's essential, therefore, for the clinician to obtain information from you, as a parent, and from your daughter's teachers. Frankly, a one-on-one interaction in an office can leave ADHD undetected, particularly if the clinician believes that unless your daughter is running around the waiting room before the appointment starts, she couldn't possibly have ADHD. Unlike anxiety or depression, for which the individual can tell the clinician about the core internal feelings and symptoms, ADHD is diagnosed chiefly on the basis of behaviors in the everyday world.

At the same time, this chapter will reveal what needs to be done to make a *differential diagnosis* (that is, what's ADHD and what's something else) as well as an *additional diagnosis* (that is, a comorbid condition that accompanies ADHD).

It's crucial to keep in mind that all of us—males and females, kids and adults—lie at various points on the dual spectra of inattentive and hyperactive-impulsive behavioral patterns. When these patterns cause real trouble is a matter of *degree,* not of sheer presence or absence. Even more, making the diagnostic determination requires an accurate sense of how much, and in what ways, the core tendencies and patterns truly interfere with school, life at home, peer interactions, self-esteem, and many other areas of functioning.

The point at which symptoms interfere with functioning can also vary widely among individuals. Looking at depression, for example, some of us are pretty optimistic despite life's ups and downs, but others are more perennially gloomy and negative. Making a clinical decision as to where, on the pessimistic and unmotivated side, everyday sadness leaves off and major depression begins requires a lot of information about the individual—about not only the depth and degree of such symptoms but also how much they get in the way of key life functions for that person.

For the most part, I focus in this chapter on procedures that are considered "ideal"—that is, the kinds of evidence-based assessments that have the best chance of identifying what's ADHD and what's not. Yet too many nonspecialist practitioners and clinicians are either not familiar with or not qualified for such an undertaking. And even if the clinician is "in the know," getting reimbursed for a full assessment can be a real challenge. Furthermore, even some of the better clinicians out there may not fully be in tune with the issues involved in evaluating ADHD in girls.

As a result, it really pays off to talk with local families, with support/advocacy groups, or with your daughter's general pediatrician about those practitioners and clinicians in your area who know how to make an accurate diagnosis of ADHD in girls. Such professionals do not diagnose everyone who enters the clinic as having ADHD—yet they also do not cling to the old-school belief that ADHD is not really a "girl" thing.

Let me be clear on what you do *not* want: a clinician who spends a brief 15-minute office visit, perhaps taking measures of your daughter's height and weight and holding an ultrabrief discussion with you about her home and school behavior, without having you and the teacher(s) complete rating scales (and, ideally, talking directly with her school). Or a professional who fails to get a sense of your daughter's early years through a careful and detailed interview with you—or who ends the all-too-brief session by pulling out a prescription pad after making an ultraquick diagnosis.

Finally, avoid clinicians who don't understand the sometimes subtle but all-too-real manifestations of ADHD in girls, who insist that only boylike dangerous and impulsive behavior patterns qualify for a

A proper evaluation takes time. Beware the "quick and dirty" assessment.

diagnosis. In all, cursory assessments made on the basis of male standards are simply not sufficient, for reasons that will become apparent as this chapter unfolds.

Should Your Daughter Be Evaluated at School or by an Outside Clinician?

Following is a brief review of the kinds of professionals in your communities whom you might ask to determine whether an ADHD diagnosis is correct for your daughter. But you may be wondering first whether your daughter should be evaluated by her school or by an outside clinician. After all, ADHD-related problems often show up at school, and the impetus for getting an evaluation in the first place may be coming from your daughter's teachers as much as from you. (Note that this is particularly true for boys and may be less the case for some girls, especially if the major concern is inattention rather than disruptive behavior; see Chapter 1.)

Your daughter may be eligible to receive accommodations and special services at school if any academic struggles your daughter is experiencing are related to ADHD (or a number of other underlying conditions). There are two types of federal statutes designed to assist individuals with disabilities. One program is called a 504 plan (under section 504 of the Federal Civil Rights Act of 1973); the other is an individualized education program under the Individuals with Disabilities Education Act (see Chapter 7, the Resources section at the end of this book, and *https://additudemag.com/iep-step-5-evaluate-your-options* for more information on both).

Whether you or your child's teacher initiates an investigation at school about why your daughter is struggling, you should request a teacher conference and present notes on your daughter's behavior and grades. At that time, the school reports on her behavior and academic performance. Those initial steps may be followed by a school-based evaluation of your daughter's ADHD and underlying learning issues. It's on the basis of such an assessment that the qualification for accommodations will be determined.

But if you wait for the school psychologist or other professionals involved with the school district to perform this evaluation, they may not focus on ADHD as much as you believe necessary—and a denial of accommodations can be likely. Thus, a clear recommendation from many experts and advocates is that you have your daughter clinically evaluated *as* you begin to request services and accommodations. The report generated from that evaluation may be extremely important. Of course, limited availability of skilled clinicians, and costs of this evaluation, need to be considered. Here's where it's important to know who is qualified to do what regarding an ADHD evaluation of your daughter.

Don't wait: Seek a clinical evaluation when you begin to ask for school accommodations.

There's a chance that the school may not "rely" on outside expert evaluations in terms of accommodations, but it certainly can't hurt to initiate an evidence-based assessment.

Who's Who in the Clinical World?

If you are seeking a clinical evaluation outside of your daughter's school, the following are the professionals you may encounter. If your child is being evaluated only at school, the evaluator will probably be a school psychologist, often in collaboration with other specialists (a speech and language expert and the like).

Medical Doctors

On the medical side, for children and adolescents, are *pediatricians,* trained in diseases of young people. They provide regular medical checkups during your child's early years but often do not have any specialty training in attention-related, behavioral, or learning disorders. For adults, the counterpart would be *general practitioners (GPs)*—or, with some additional training, *family practitioners* who are qualified to work with family members of all ages.

All of them are medical doctors (MDs), who have gone to medical school and can prescribe medications for a range of physical and mental conditions. Although levels of training and experience vary, most are not experts in ADHD, especially in girls.

There are a small number of more specialized pediatricians, called *developmental/behavioral pediatricians,* who have spent extra years in training to study learning, behavioral, and attention-related issues in young people. If there were more of these specialists around, they would be priorities for assessment of your daughter.

Another medical specialization is psychiatry. *Child and adolescent psychiatrists* are medical doctors who spend additional years after their basic psychiatry training to learn about behavioral, attentional, and emotional issues in young people. Another medical specialty is neurology. Neurologists are experts in brain diseases. Thus, they are sometimes called in to assist in diagnosing ADHD, especially if their training has been in child neurology and if there's an issue in distinguishing ADHD from, for example, a head injury or a seizure.

All doctors have extensive training in the medical model. But they may not be as well versed in the appraisal of behavior patterns at home and school as they are in basic biological processes. The specialists noted above (developmental/behavioral pediatricians or child/adolescent psychiatrists) are typically more familiar with and skilled in proper evaluations regarding ADHD. Again, though, their numbers are few, especially outside of major urban areas, and it may take a very long time to get an appointment with them.

Psychologists

Next are psychologists, particularly those who have received a doctoral degree in clinical or school psychology. These *clinical or school psychologists* cannot prescribe medications, except in a very few locations, but they are typically trained in the kinds of rating scales, interviews, and tests that can help to pinpoint a diagnosis of ADHD, with or without additional conditions. Some clinical psychologists specialize in adults, rather than children; and not all psychologists (either clinical or school) have specialization in what it takes to diagnose ADHD. Yet those who do can often work in real partnership with medical doctors not only to diagnose ADHD but also to treat it from multiple angles.

Neuropsychologists are doctoral-level psychologists who specialize in the intricate kinds of one-on-one tests that can help to identify perceptual (visual, auditory), cognitive (reading, math, basic language), and "executive" (planning, working memory, inhibition) processes that can generate a fine-grained picture of your daughter's cognitive strengths and weaknesses. Please note that such neuropsychological testing can be exceedingly expensive. Even more, the diagnosis of ADHD is based far more on observable behavior than on underlying cognitive deficits. Nonetheless, a thorough neuropsychological evaluation may help you and your family begin to disentangle language/learning/perceptual issues from ADHD-related issues, especially for complex cases—as noted later in this chapter.

Master's-Level Clinicians

Most counselors, marriage and family therapists, and social workers have a master's degree. Such individuals, along with "coaches" (who for the most part are not formally certified), may be valuable for some families of girls with ADHD, or for adults with ADHD, especially with respect to family support or, in the case of school social workers, school support. Yet unless they are exceptionally well trained and work in conjunction with medical doctors and psychologists, they are typically not properly educated in the assessment and diagnosis of ADHD.

The Bottom Line

I must admit: If you have found it confusing to understand the array of professionals just discussed, along with their academic degrees and their associated levels of skill, I have too! But my hope is that this brief orientation can help you understand which kinds of professionals may be most helpful. Do not rely on guesswork. Instead, do as much research as you can regarding the best options in your area.

Look for the best-qualified specialist(s) in your area to have your daughter evaluated.

What Are You Seeing in Your Daughter?

What impressions and observations are leading you to request a clinical assessment? You could be the parent of a really troublesome preschool-age girl whose disruptive behavior patterns have her teachers—and her peers, and the parents of those peers—perplexed and even afraid of her erratic behavior. She can't sit still, she won't (or can't) follow directions, she lashes out at anyone trying to set limits, and she may even be engaging in dangerous behavior patterns. Her career in kindergarten and later grades could be at real risk. In such a case it's clear-cut: Getting an evaluation as soon as you can is essential.

But for most parents, things are (or were) not this extreme at the age of 3 or 4. Yes, issues may well be tough, in that your daughter may display subtle language or cognitive issues or might not fit as well into her peer group as you'd hoped. Somehow the family has managed, even if, at times, barely. During the elementary-school years, your daughter may seem less eager and willing than her siblings or her peers to engage in academics. Her levels of effort appear sporadic. She may have trouble lasting through a whole meal with the family, to say nothing of a homework session. Her moodiness or trouble maintaining focus may throw the whole family off-kilter. In fact, her siblings may be wondering why she gets such attention, positive and (mainly) negative, from you.

As discussed in Chapter 1, girls have a greater likelihood than boys do of showing the exclusively (or largely) inattentive form of ADHD. So, your daughter may not be as overtly impulsive as most boys who show ADHD symptoms: She may not be throwing spit wads in class or engaging in overtly risky behavior at home. Still, other indicators can drive you to distraction. For example, she may argue over every request, constantly leave her room and belongings an utter mess, seem not to listen when you give her the same requests over (and over), or interrupt you or family friends to the point of embarrassment (for you, not necessarily for her).

Alternatively, she may appear withdrawn, disorganized, a bit lonely, and in her own world. The demands of home and school life seem to overwhelm her. Somehow, when you try to talk with her about these kinds of issues, you can't seem to reach her: She's defensive, ashamed, angry, or just shut down. (More details about identifying ADHD in young girls can be found in Chapter 8.)

Moving forward in terms of development, there may be big issues during the transition to middle school. Somehow, you now realize, she eked by during elementary school with decent (or semidecent, or even excellent) grades and a semitypical home life, but it took *so* much structuring on your part to get her there. Was it the dragging her to tutors or after-school programs? Helping her a lot (maybe even too much) with homework? Rushing frantically to get to school or appointments on time—with much of it a constant struggle? Seeing that formerly happy daughter of yours slowly get more demoralized with each year of school—and especially so now, when the double risk of puberty and middle school arise at the same time?

The transition to high school can be equally challenging, as the work gets ever more difficult and the demands for organization and independence intensify.

In other words, the self-regulation problems underlying ADHD come to the fore, all too often, when new developmental challenges occur and when your family's efforts just can't seem to match the new contexts and expectations your daughter is experiencing.

What Are Your Daughter's Teachers Seeing in Her?

In most assessments for ADHD, it's the impressions of *teachers* that begin to push the family to consider a diagnosis. Especially if your daughter is an only child—or if she has brothers but not sisters—you may not realize that the daily struggles you're encountering are a sign of an underlying clinical issue. Yet your daughter's teacher is the one who may well be saying, at a parent–teacher conference or in an unexpected e-mail or school portal message to you (with the subject line marked "urgent"), that she's not thriving the way she could be.

Other examples of such feedback might pierce your heart: Teachers may report that they either can't abide your daughter's unruly behavior or can't bear to see what seems like self-sabotage—not completing assignments, claiming she can't find her homework, not hearing the repeated instructions to do things a certain way. They may give, as well, the more general sense that she's just not living up to her potential . . . she's acting far younger than her chronological age . . . her emotions seem out of check too much of the time. Or, she's digging herself into a corner because, although she knows what she's supposed to do, she just can't consistently apply herself to meet those standards. Her inattentive and impulsive behaviors are interfering not just with her own learning but with the learning of her classmates.

If your daughter is on the more exclusively inattentive end of the spectrum, teachers are likely to voice their concerns in terms of low motivation, her being "lost" in the crowd, or simply underperforming in school, especially when the work gets more challenging.

All such observations may shake your implicit belief that if she just matures enough, she'll finally be out of the woods. Or that your intensive coping efforts can save the day if you just soldier on.

Other school-related indicators may be as simple as examining her report card: Does she show a range of grades, across different classes, from A to D or F—the consistent inconsistency mentioned in Chapter 1? Do her teachers lament that if she could only "get organized" everything would be fine? Or do they seem to be questioning what on earth may be going on at home to prompt her inconsistent, frustrating, and sometimes maddening behaviors? All this feedback can impose a heavy burden on you and the family, but a really good evaluation can be the first step toward needed help.

Initial Conversations with a Clinician

Sooner or later, you may come to the following realizations regarding your daughter:

> *These issues are not likely to go away of their own accord.*
> *It's time that we get a handle on what's getting in the way of her thriving—and even our family's sanity.*
> *We need to find someone who can give us some clear answers.*

As you research ways of managing that requested parent–teacher conference and then finding out who's the best clinician for an evaluation, you'll want to consider what your initial "statement" should entail. My advice: Get as organized as you can in putting together your and your family's impressions. These may have been building for many years. They may also have been propelled by a recent crisis—such as your daughter's being sent to the principal's office or failing a class—or the revelation that the perceptions of teachers, neighbors, and other girls, as well as your own growing impressions, are not getting any better. Your daughter herself may be getting so demoralized and confused over what's going wrong that she actually wants some help.

While you compose the e-mail or prepare for the initial conversation, collect report cards, "diaries" or notes of your concerns, past health records (immunizations, accidents, head injuries, any hospitalizations, tutoring, special services received), and impressions of earlier professional visits, if there are any. From these raw materials, write out an outline, which could include answers to the following questions:

- What are the patterns you've been observing over the past months (or years)? Sure, you're confused, upset, and even impatient at this point, but try to lay out a brief timeline of the origins of your concerns. Patterns may emerge that you hadn't noted before.
- What are key examples of your daughter's inattentiveness, lack of self-regulation, and/or impulsivity—at home, in school, with peers?

- Which teachers, or other educational or health care providers, have made comments to you? What's the substance of their concerns? Are there certain school subjects that are consistently more difficult for your daughter than others? Alternatively, in which kinds of classrooms or other situations has she relatively thrived?

- How has your family's life been affected?

The computer file or even paper file of the materials you've collected, along with your outline, can help you organize and streamline the forthcoming assessment process. They should give the assessor something to chew on, initially, over and above what might seem to be the complaints of yet another distraught parent. Finally, they should help with the many questions that a thorough evaluator will have for you.

The preceding can help you provide what the evaluator will need to make the most accurate assessment possible. But it's also wise for you to enter the process with realistic expectations and an open mind. As you get closer to the evaluation, keep the following in mind:

- A number of other issues can look at lot like ADHD, including neurological problems (like some kinds of seizures or the aftereffects of head injuries), maltreatment, chronic stress, depression, anxiety, or chaotic classrooms. Or real family stress.

- And even when diagnosed well, ADHD is often accompanied by additional learning, emotional, and/or behavioral problems, which may need additional treatments.

- The moral: Rome was not built in a day. ADHD cannot be evaluated accurately in a single, brief office visit. Prepare for some soul-searching, on your daughter's part (depending on how old she is), on your part, and on the whole family's part, as you come to terms with what the core of the problem might be and with the kinds of changes that may need to be made at home and at school.

An evaluation for ADHD can be a long haul. It's time well spent, for your daughter's sake.

Now, what should you expect from the formal evaluation process?

The Evaluation Process: Diving Deeper

I've said it before, but I'll say it again: The core information needed to make a diagnosis of ADHD in a child or adolescent comes not from an intensive, one-on-one interview with the youth in question but from observations of her behavior in everyday settings. One of the best ways of obtaining such information comes from rating scales, completed by parents and separately by teachers, about your daughter's behavior at home and at school.

Rating Scales/Checklists

An excellent way for the clinician to get important information is by asking you, and your daughter's teacher(s), to complete one or more standardized rating scales—sometimes called "checklists" or "questionnaires"—about her typical behavior patterns. There are huge advantages to doing so, as no clinician, except in a well-funded research study, can afford the time (nor can you afford the cost) of having hidden video cameras or live observers in rooms of your home or in your daughter's classroom, to record daily behaviors related to ADHD or other conditions. Just think of the logistical and even ethical issues here, too. Even more, with such minute-by-minute accounts, who would summarize and score all of the behavioral information? A checklist, however, can be completed in a relatively brief amount of time.

After an initial call explaining the evaluation process, the clinician should send you and your daughter's teacher, by mail or electronically, the scale(s), having each of you separately complete them before the evaluation continues. In this way, the clinician can get a good sense of behavioral tendencies, both at home and at school, which can help to guide the rest of the diagnostic procedures and the eventual treatment plan.

There are two types of behavioral rating scales. "Narrow" scales consist of the lists of ADHD symptoms that make up the official diagnostic criteria, or perhaps a few additional items. "Broad" and more inclusive scales include many more items related to a whole range of behavioral and emotional issues, such as anxious behavior, depression, and aggression.

The shorter ADHD-only checklists can be completed in a couple of minutes. They can help begin an assessment and are especially useful during periods of trying out ADHD medications or behavioral treatments, to see whether change is occurring.

The broad, comprehensive checklists have the distinct advantage of informing the clinician (and you) about additional problem areas your daughter may be experiencing. Yet some of them contain over 100 items and involve a more substantial time investment of 15–20 minutes or longer.

How Do They Work?

Core examples of narrow and broad rating scales/checklists appear in Resources, at the end of the book, under "Assessment and Diagnosis." For such scales, the parent or teacher rates each item (for example, "shows difficulty in paying attention") on a quantitative scale like the following:

0—not at all
1—just a little
2—pretty much
3—very much

The instructions also include a time frame within which parents or teachers make their rating. Some narrow scales might specify "today" (and these can be really helpful for detecting medication effects on a day-by-day basis), but most will include a time period ranging from the past week to the past month—or even the past six months.

Again, parents complete their version of the scale and teachers their own version (items may differ slightly given the different nature of home settings and school environments). The clinician then scores items according to the numerical rating for each, to get a total score related to inattention and hyperactivity/impulsivity—or, for the more comprehensive scales, areas like defiance, fears, peer problems, depression, and many more.

Norms

Beyond the ability of the assessor to "see" home and school behavior patterns from these checklists, there's another huge advantage. During the construction of each scale, the authors made sure that thousands of parents and thousands of teachers completed the ratings. So, your daughter's scores can be compared directly to those of many other girls in her age bracket. In other words, there is a built-in comparison to see how far she scores above the average of other youth at the same age. There is a debate among experts about whether the comparison should be made with just other girls of her age or with both boys and girls; see the box below.

As an example, the assessor can see that a particular fifth grader has a primary teacher who rates her as being in the 98th percentile of all girls her age with respect to inattention—far above average!—but only the 54th percentile with respect to hyperactivity/impulsivity, which is in the middle of the distribution. In this hypothetical case, let's assume that the parents provide essentially the same pattern of scores. The clinician can therefore provide the family with guidance regarding not only whether ADHD symptoms are extreme but also which form or presentation of ADHD is most likely—in this case, the inattentive form.

Should Girls Be Compared with Girls or Both Boys and Girls?

A question that's actively debated among ADHD experts is whether, regarding rating scales/questionnaires gathered from parents and teachers, the girl should be "scored" in relation to (1) all youth (boys and girls) of her age or (2) only girls in her age bracket.

In the general population, boys score higher than girls, especially on hyperactivity/impulsivity. So, comparing a girl to both boys and girls makes it more difficult for her to end up in the clinical range. If she is compared only to girls—that is, with a "lower bar"—she may more readily qualify for an ADHD diagnosis.

If we immediately went to sex-specific norms, more girls would clearly qualify for a diagnosis. But would lowering the bar in this way be valid? Consider the case for depression in men. It is well known that, around the world, in adolescence and beyond, girls and women have double (or more) the rates of major depression of boys and men. Does that mean that we automatically start judging the latter on the basis of norms from other males? Doing so would clearly make rates of diagnosis far closer to equal in men and women, but just as with ADHD, it's not clear that males would truly have the same levels of impairment as men meeting the more stringent sex-general norms.

I do believe that sex differences (both biological and those culturally based) produce different rates of mental and learning issues between the sexes. So, using sex-specific norms simply to equalize rates between the sexes is not, in my view, what we should automatically do.

But what if the parents and teachers don't agree all that much? The evaluator then needs to probe further to understand your daughter's behaviors in specific contexts.

What if your daughter is in middle school or high school: Does the assessor need to get a rating scale from each of her five or six teachers? That would be asking a lot, for sure. One way to handle this situation is to request the rating scale from one teacher in math or science and another in language arts. Or one with whom your daughter seems to have real problems and another with whom she's perhaps a better fit.

Note: If your daughter is beyond the preschool years, a skilled assessor may ask you to help obtain rating scales from not only this year's teacher(s) but also last year's or even earlier. Why? The answer is that ADHD behavior patterns vary from year to year in different classrooms. In other words, how your daughter "fits" in her current classroom with her current teacher may not be the same as that "fit" in previous years. It's almost like the rings of a large tree: Your daughter may have had, frankly, a hellish time in kindergarten, first grade, and second grade—but then in third grade, her teacher somehow "got" her, understood her attentional and learning differences, and at the same time helped her thrive. Then, sadly, her fourth and fifth grade teachers weren't as sensitive or flexible. If the assessor can view that pattern, it may not only help with the diagnosis of ADHD but also assist in finding the kinds of strategies that may help with intervention planning for the future.

What about Reports from Your Daughter?

In the stereotypical view of how psychological and educational assessments happen, there's often a magical scene in which asking the key questions of the person being evaluated leads to a revelation. At last, the individual understands the core problem and we can now move on from there to a brighter future!

But except in rare instances, this isn't the case for ADHD in children and adolescents (or even adults). Recall from Chapter 1 that the core "attentional" problem in ADHD isn't just a lack of sustained attention to rote or challenging tasks but instead a problem with the *regulation* of attention across a task, a school period, or a day. Such inconsistent attention may also pertain to your daughter's views of herself. To make a long story short, especially for children and adolescents with ADHD, there's a common tendency for them to underreport their levels of problematic attention and behavior. Rather than openly acknowledging problems in following directions, completing tasks, and restraining impulses, people (including girls) with ADHD may direct the blame outward, not just out of denial or defensiveness but also from a lack of recognition of how they may contribute to the process and problems.

> *That teacher has it in for me.*
> *My friends don't understand what I want.*
> *My parents hassle me all the time that I'm not living up to their ideals—why don't they just get who I am?*

The bottom line is that although children with depression or anxiety can often be good reporters on their own issues in these domains—in fact, probably the optimal reporters—children with attention- and impulse-related problems are typically *not* optimal informants on those very issues. Although a child with ADHD must be a part of the evaluation process, especially regarding information about their sense of self-worth, their goals, their fears, and their possible self-recriminations, their input with respect to the core symptoms of ADHD is typically limited. By adolescence, however, they may be more self-aware (though often not completely).

In sum, adult reporters, particularly parents and teachers, should "carry the day" in terms of the most important information about the youth's ADHD-related issues. Getting the girl's input is still vital, especially regarding her engagement in ongoing treatment, but her self-report of ADHD behaviors must give way to accounts from adult informants.

> *Reports from your daughter about her experiences with ADHD symptoms are usually not helpful for making a diagnosis. Rely on yourself and teachers for more accurate information.*

Are Parents and Teachers Perfect Informants?

The short answer is no. In fact, no single source of information is infallible in any assessment process.

Let's look at parent reports on rating scales. Perhaps your daughter is your only child: How much do you really know about what to expect from an elementary-school-age or middle school girl at home? Cultural values can certainly play a role, too: Certain cultures that value child obedience and strict adherence to adult norms may see everyday child disgruntlement, or a bid for independence, as hugely atypical, inflating parental ratings.

In parallel, some teachers value order and control above all else, so that any girl who deviates even slightly from such standards may be viewed as a huge problem. Yet other teachers, perhaps in underfunded school districts or those with a high rate of students with histories of abuse, may have developed a high tolerance for attentional lapses or impulse-control problems, failing to actively notice a girl with true attention deficits.

The core point is that the clinician should not just obtain ratings but, when possible, observe home and school behavior to the greatest extent possible, and synthesize information from adult ratings with developmental interviews and testing results (see next section).

Here's a final—and important—issue related to interpreting scores on rating scales, especially from teachers. If you end up getting a look at such school-based ratings, you may wonder why, in some cases, the teacher doesn't seem to be reporting the problems and issues you know your daughter has been experiencing for some time. Well, maybe this particular teacher knows your daughter well enough—and is on sufficient lookout for her well-being—that the teacher provides extra supports and "coaching" that actually serve to minimize impairment and problems at school. For example, the teacher may repeat instructions for your daughter and provide extra reminders. If this is the case, it would be important for you, and the clinician, to ask the teacher what those ratings would look like in the absence of such supports.

The same might apply to your own ratings: Perhaps you've provided enough special structure and guidance yourself that it's not representative of how your daughter might behave and perform in a less structured setting. The bottom line is that rating scales and questionnaires aren't just the "numbers" of scores on ADHD-related or other scales. They're actually the source of additional questions and issues about where the problems may reside.

Developmental Interviews

Next, the assessor needs to talk with you, as a parent, about a number of historical and background issues related to your daughter, as well as current strengths and weaknesses and the current family situation. That is, ADHD is not an in-the-moment diagnosis; it requires examination of behavior, cognitive, language-related, and emotion-linked issues over the course of your daughter's development. At the same time, past or current stressors at home can lead to, or keep in place, symptoms quite similar to ADHD; these also need to be considered.

A *developmental interview* is one in which the clinician asks you about your daughter's lifelong patterns of behavior, as well as the family's and school's responses. Before such an interview, it helps to collect records from her birth, if you are the biological parent (or to search for records available if you are not). Pregnancy-related or "perinatal"—that is, right around the time of her birth—issues may also be clues. Collecting records from her pediatrician, notes you wrote down during her early years, or even scrapbooks or cell-phone photos could help to recall when she turned over, crawled, walked, and began to talk. And subsequently, how her language developed. You can also note how she began to interact and play with peers, and what her reactions were to her first child-care workers and teachers.

Sometimes the clinician may actually send you an open-ended questionnaire with some of these questions. Even then, it's important to have time to review and discuss your written responses with the assessor and to elaborate on them.

All this is important because ADHD does not exist in a vacuum. Subtle problems in your daughter's motor development, delays in her speech and language, early interactions with other caregivers, or traumatic events she may have experienced can be associated with ADHD and serve as a signal that other clinical issues are present. Even if life stressors in your family did not cause her ADHD symptoms, they could be maintaining or exacerbating them.

A word of caution: If the evaluation doesn't leave time for such questions and answers, be suspicious.

Testing

Now that the assessor has information on your daughter's current and past functioning at home and school, and on her levels of attention and impulsive behavior compared to other girls her age, what else can aid with the evaluation?

First, there's the key question of how accurate your ratings, and the teacher's ratings, really are. That is, how representative is your home—or your daughter's classroom—of other homes and schools around the country?

Maybe your impressions, or those of her teacher, are the product of other factors. Even in families with lots of love, raising a daughter with the symptoms of ADHD can lead to considerable family stress, as discussed at more length in later chapters. As a result, you may be experiencing increasingly negative attitudes about your daughter—and so might her teacher(s). On the other hand, if she's viewed as compliant and generally nice, perhaps the ratings aren't really picking up on some of her core underlying problems. Isn't there a more objective measure for diagnosing ADHD?

Computerized Tests of Attention

By now, a number of test publishers have produced computerized measures of an individual's ability to maintain focus on, or refrain from distractions related to, tests of performance on standardized measures of attention. These might seem to be a great solution: Rather than rely on parent and teacher reports—or the hard-to-attain observations of your daughter's performance at school—perhaps we finally have an objective way of observing her attentional capacities.

For example, on a laptop or desktop computer screen, she might be asked to push a certain key if she sees the letters A/B/C/D/E but a different key if she sees F/G/H/I/J. The longer the test goes on and the more that fatigue may set in, the more errors she is likely to make. A person's responses to such objective tests are not subject to the vagaries of particular homes or school settings, or even to various clinicians' offices. These assessments might therefore yield a measure of *sustained attention* or *freedom from distraction* less prone to an observer's bias.

Yet consider this: How well does your daughter's performance on a supposedly objective computerized test compare to her performance in a busy classroom? Or at home, with parents, siblings, and even pets competing for her (and your) attention? Research reveals that an individual's scores on such one-on-one tests are influenced by whether the assessor is sitting next to them or they're left alone. Even though boys and girls with ADHD do worse, on average, on such tests than do those without ADHD, many with ADHD actually do quite well in the idealized situation of such individualized computer tests. In short, test performance may not predict her actions in the real world with enough accuracy; these tests are not as objective or accurate as was once believed. Computerized tests of attention can help the clinician by adding data to the assessment, but they cannot substitute for the appraisal of your daughter's behaviors at home or in the classroom.

Tests of Intelligence, Academic Achievement, and Neuropsychological Performance

Giving an individually administered IQ test was once thought to be crucial for making a diagnosis of ADHD. Over and above the total IQ score, different patterns of performance across the different subtests were thought to indicate an underlying index consistent with ADHD. Although tests of intelligence can be useful for understanding strengths and weaknesses in overall cognitive abilities, just like computerized tests of attention, IQ test performance under idealized circumstances may not correspond well to your daughter's performance in a classroom setting, with all of the noise and distractions going on. In addition, studies have also largely dispelled the notion that a certain profile of subtest scores can precisely pinpoint ADHD.

Regarding achievement, tests of reading and math are essential for assessing the presence of learning disorders. It's clearly important to know your daughter's academic proficiency in basic academic subjects. But like the other one-on-one tests just noted, they are not sufficient to make a clear diagnosis of ADHD in your daughter. They can be most useful for academic planning and to obtain a more complete picture of her abilities. But don't count on them to make an ADHD diagnosis.

Neuropsychological tests refer to those batteries of one-on-one measures that a neuropsychologist gives to someone suspected of having learning, attentional, or related issues. Like some of the subtests of an overall IQ measure, they aim to pinpoint issues in memory, perception, attention, visual abilities, and auditory abilities, as well as core executive functions (planning, subtle problems with impulse control, resistance to distraction, working memory, and more). There are a large number of such tests, which can be valuable for understanding the cognitive abilities of individuals who have experienced head injuries, who have had a stroke, or who are starting to show signs of dementia. The question is whether they are necessary for a diagnosis of ADHD.

A neuropsychological evaluation is rarely needed to diagnose ADHD and can be prohibitively expensive.

As you might suspect from the preceding paragraphs, no one-on-one test can accurately represent the individual's performance in the real world. Even more, the costs of obtaining a complete neuropsychological evaluation for your daughter can be staggering.

If your clinician says that the only way to diagnose ADHD is through a lengthy neuropsychological battery, don't believe it. On the one hand, there may be complicated processes, in your daughter, spanning attentional, learning, trauma-related, and injury-linked issues. If you can afford (or find coverage for) the relevant costs, neuropsychological testing could be indicated as part of a truly complete evaluation. On the other hand, diagnosing ADHD does not usually require the lengthy testing and expenses linked with a full neuropsychological battery.

Brain Scans

Over the past few decades, revolutionary advances have emerged in the ability to observe the brain both at rest and in the performance of complex cognitive tasks. You may encounter mention of (or recommendations for) CT scans, MRIs and fMRIs, EEGs, PET scans, and SPECT scans. In some ways, these scans have been the holy grail: At last, now available is a completely objective means of diagnosing ADHD—and a number of other mental and neurodevelopmental conditions—on the basis of actual "pictures" of the brain in action.

Despite the promise, please don't rush to the nearest neuroimaging center. Yes, the science of brain-based activities that relate to ADHD is advancing. Issues in the frontal lobes, and their intricate interconnections with multiple other brain regions, underlie dysregulated attention, poor response inhibition, and many more functions linked with ADHD. But there is no single "brain signature" of ADHD at present, nor is there likely to be one anytime soon. As discussed in Chapter 1, there are a host of genetic vulnerabilities, their interactions with early-life environments and with home and school contexts, plus related motivational factors that can combine to yield what we now call ADHD. In fact, it is probable that ADHD will turn out to constitute a variety of conditions with shared symptoms, each

> *ADHD remains a "low-tech" diagnosis—don't expect to get specific answers from expensive brain imaging.*

of which displays different risk factors and combinations thereof, which remain beyond our comprehension until the science advances.

We are simply not at the stage of having a definitive diagnosis of ADHD based on the results of brain imaging, no matter what you may read on websites or hear from social media posts. Don't believe anyone who tells you—at the potential cost of thousands of dollars—that a SPECT scan, for example, can give you a magic ticket into understanding your daughter's underlying brain patterns and yield a precise treatment plan. ADHD remains a "low-tech" diagnosis for the time being, requiring a careful synthesis of impressions from parents, teachers, and after-school personnel, with a thorough account of developmental history and information from individual assessments. There is no way that any single source can make it all happen.

Medical Screening

Your pediatrician should have been collecting information since infancy about your daughter's height and weight and about her speech, motor, and other developmental milestones. Beyond such basic measures, are there other medical evaluations that can pinpoint ADHD?

No, not really. Again, ADHD diagnoses are made on the basis of behaviors, not blood tests, brain scans, or tissue samples. Yet there are physical issues and conditions that need to be either taken into account or "ruled out" when establishing an ADHD diagnosis.

• *Screening for vision and hearing.* If your daughter can't see or hear well, she may not be able to concentrate on written materials or follow spoken directions (which she's not able to process). For the latter, chronic ear infections might be playing a role.

• *Brief neurological examination.* This is not a brain scan but instead a doctor's brief, office-based examination of basic sensory functions, alertness, core memory, and the like. If your daughter has problematic functioning on this screening, further referral to a neurologist may be in order, as there could be other conditions underlying what appear to be symptoms of ADHD.

• *Rule-outs.* First, if there are questions of an underlying seizure disorder, a neurological consultation is clearly in order. In fact, certain types of "minor" seizures involved brief periods of inattentiveness. Second, thyroid issues can underlie ADHD symptoms in certain cases. Third, sleep problems are important to consider: Overtiredness can certainly lead to concentration problems, as we all know. Furthermore, ADHD (and its many comorbid accompaniments) may predict problems with sleep. Fourth, levels of toxic chemicals (such as lead) in the bloodstream can contribute to ADHD symptoms and poor learning. In fact, lead levels well below those typically considered "lead poisoning" can still be contributors. Fifth, has your daughter had a head injury? Symptoms of concussion can clearly include poor concentration—and it is now known that youth with ADHD are more prone to head injuries and concussions than other young people.

• *Cardiac screening.* A doctor who is considering a trial of ADHD medication may order a heart screening test, such as an electrocardiogram (EKG). Especially for individuals with known heart anomalies or family histories of heart disease, stimulant medications may trigger overstimulation of the heart. After close study, medical expert panels have not deemed such screenings necessary for everyone who is a candidate for ADHD medications. The costs of these screenings are too high, and the rates of cardiac issues related to the medications in question are quite low. Still, you may be asked to provide information on your daughter and your family members regarding any history of heart-related issues—and in some cases, an EKG may be ordered.

Specific Issues in Assessing Girls with Suspected ADHD

The following considerations can be just as important as completing the appropriate rating scales, giving a sound developmental history, and obtaining tests and medical screening.

Not Just Symptoms but Impairment

Official guides to diagnosis contend, rightfully, that it's not just a set number of symptoms that indicate the presence of ADHD but (1) their presence in at least two settings (such as home, school, and peer group) and (2) the levels of life functioning that they compromise. So don't be surprised if the clinician asks your daughter questions relating to how she feels about herself, her beliefs about how her teachers and you feel about her, and her perceptions of how she gets along with peers in class and in the neighborhood. For teens, romantic relationships would be open for discussion as well. The clinician should also be probing you about your daughter's academic performance, the patterns of family interactions that typically exist at home, your perceptions of how she gets along with other adults and her peer group, accidental injuries she might have experienced, and more.

It's also quite important to obtain information about her skills and strengths. When your car gets tuned up, the mechanic may point out that the brake pads and spark plugs need replacing—but almost never comments on how well the transmission is working. But your daughter, I hasten to add, is not a car!

People's competencies and strong points can help to outweigh and overcome particular weaknesses that may be revealed in an evidence-based evaluation. In fact, as I emphasize strongly in Chapters 8 and 9, it's essential to seek and nurture those activities that your daughter loves and prioritizes. These can provide important rewards for the behavioral program you build—and may even end up as important steps in her push toward both independence and connection later in life. Make sure that you come away from the assessment with a report that conveys your daughter's strong points as well as her particular weaknesses.

> *Strengths are just as important for an assessment to reveal as weaknesses.*

Bias in ADHD Scales and Interviews

Even if your clinician uses state-of-the-art rating scales and developmental interviews, it can still be the case that male-dominated ADHD items on such measures prevent too many girls (and women) from receiving an accurate diagnosis. As discussed in Chapter 1, when evaluating females, it is essential to emphasize (1) the inattentive and disorganized symptoms of ADHD and (2) more subtle kinds of impulsivity and hyperactivity. Also, it could be the case that your clinician still holds to the old-school mentality that ADHD does not exist in girls. You'll never know unless you ask directly. If so, be on the lookout for a different clinician.

Overachievement and Overcompensation

Recall from Chapter 1 that a number of girls who have ADHD may be masking the relevant symptoms because they are strongly concerned with "doing well." Their tendencies to overworry, overstudy, and overcompensate can give the false appearance that everything is fine. But there's a major cost to your daughter's perfectionism in terms of growing stress levels—and the inevitable crash when the workload gets so hard that no amount of overcompensation can pull her out of the fire. It may also be that massive family supports are preventing her ADHD symptoms and impairments from coming to the fore. In short, beyond counts of symptoms per se, the assessor needs to ask about your daughter's compensatory strategies and the family's "support network," which may be covering over her underlying issues.

Assessments at Different Ages

As girls (and boys) suspected of having ADHD get older, they mature (even if at a relatively slow rate), their home and school environments change, expectations for performance get ever more demanding, and their worlds widen. All this means that evaluations for ADHD will take somewhat different forms when initiated at different ages.

For preschoolers, it's mainly the impulsive and disruptive behavior patterns that get recognition, given that the lack of a structured academic curriculum prevents detection of all but the most severe forms of inattention. It could also be tempting to prematurely diagnose a 3- or 4-year-old who is "squirrely" and hard to manage but who will improve, in a couple of years, with more structure and maturation. In order to understand truly exceptional levels of these behaviors, preschool versions of rating scales for both parents and preschool teachers should be used, with good norms, to ensure that the behaviors are truly extreme for the age.

It would be a real mistake, however, to think that ADHD cannot exist during the preschool years. Detection of the most severe presentations of ADHD at that age range could help to propel family and school intervention plans, along with other specialized services, which could help to head off growing problems and impairments throughout childhood and beyond.

The elementary-school years are the period when most ADHD diagnoses occur, at least for boys. It is then that slowed academic growth and a range of troublesome behaviors become increasingly salient at home, at school, and in the peer group.

For girls, however—especially those with predominant inattention and/ or those who are overcompensating—it may not be until middle school or high school (or even later) that accurate detection can be made. Secondary school, of course, involves high demands for organization and independent work. For the vast majority of students, it also involves having a different teacher for each class, compounding the need for excellent self-regulation (and executive functions—once again, those cognitive skills related to planning, remembering, shifting goals in midstream as needed, and correcting errors). Accordingly, assessments that focus on organizational skills and executive functioning are in order—more so than ratings or observations of fidgeting or overtly hyperactive behavior.

As your daughter enters adolescence, her own perspectives regarding her ADHD symptoms and other critical issues (like depression and anxiety, as well as coping skills) become more and more a key part of the evaluation. Self-report forms of relevant rating scales, and detailed interviews with your teenage daughter, should be explicitly included in the evaluation process.

And let's not forget that the middle school years are the time of the ascension into puberty, with the vast biological and psychosocial changes that this period entails.

Finally, sometimes ADHD doesn't get detected until the huge demands of college, the workforce, or even postcollege education are experienced. This is an important perspective to have when considering the evaluation of ADHD in women.

Assessment of Comorbid Conditions

As noted in Chapter 1, it is rare for children, adolescents, or adults with ADHD to have this diagnosis as the only one they receive. How will the clinician—and you—know whether your daughter may also be experiencing clinically significant anxiety or depression, noncompliance and/or aggression, a reaction to stress, some features of autism, or a learning disorder? Following is a brief summary of the kinds of assessment strategies that are optimal for understanding the most common associated (or comorbid) conditions.

Depression and Anxiety

Many girls with ADHD become increasingly anxious and depressed as they accumulate failure experiences during childhood. For others, particularly those with the inattentive form of ADHD, it may be hard to distinguish what's inattention versus what's anxious or depressed behavior. The clinician will need to administer parent and teacher ratings of these kinds of behavior patterns—often available from broad scales used during the initial ADHD evaluation—and directly interview your daughter herself. Anxiety and depression can respond to different forms of cognitive-behavioral therapy than is used for ADHD per se. For severe cases, different medications (especially selective serotonin reuptake inhibitors, or SSRIs)—are the medications of choice if meds are indicated.

Oppositional and Aggressive Behavior

Many girls with ADHD, whether showing the inattentive or combined presentation, get locked into battles (sometimes simmering, sometimes epic) with authority figures, like parents and teachers. This is more the case for those with the combined form of ADHD, given the impulsivity involved. Parent and teacher ratings are really important to uncover these behavior patterns, especially for preteens who may not have enough insight to recognize their role in such dysfunctional interactions. By adolescence, if your daughter becomes engaged in more serious oppositional and aggressive behavior patterns, which can include substance abuse, it's important to get her perspectives as well as yours about such issues in a thorough assessment.

PTSD

PTSD can result from natural disasters, exposure to neighborhood violence, or experiencing physical or sexual abuse. Symptoms can include a kind of shutting down, hyperresponsiveness to stimuli that serve as reminders of the trauma, and periodic reexperiencing of the trauma (nightmares, flashbacks). In younger children, many of the symptoms are consistent with anxiety, depression, and ADHD. The clinician needs to obtain information from you, the parent, and/ or records from early caregivers. It could be the case that serious trauma produces symptoms that are quite similar to ADHD symptoms. It can also be the case that early impulsivity is a risk factor for the traumatizing experiences. Furthermore, it's not either–or—as ADHD and PTSD can occur in the same youth. There's no substitute for a thorough history from the clinician to begin to sort things out.

Learning Disorders

It can be hard, in many cases, to know whether a girl has ADHD, a reading or math disorder, or both in equal measure. There's no substitute for robust reading and math testing to understand whether your daughter has a learning disorder in these areas. Furthermore, the kinds of attention problems a girl with a "pure" learning disorder displays are typically limited to time periods when she is struggling with that academic subject, whereas ADHD-related issues in attention and self-regulation typically occur in contexts well beyond academics. In all, learning disorders require focused intervention in the academic areas that are problematic, beyond ADHD-related treatments.

Autism Spectrum Disorders

Your daughter may seem extremely social, so why would the clinician be concerned with assessing behaviors that are part of the autism spectrum? In fact, some of the risk genes related to autism spectrum disorder are essentially the same as those linked with ADHD. And in some cases, the kinds of social relationship issues (as in not reading social cues well) can be shared between these conditions. As a result, the clinician may need to get additional history from you about your daughter's earliest years, her patterns of interactions with adults and peers, "odd" behaviors (such as repetitive motor and verbal actions), her potential difficulties in reading social cues, and her language abilities, which might indicate some overlap with autism spectrum behavior patterns.

In Summary

When any of these conditions accompanies ADHD, the treatment plan will need to be supplemented with condition-specific interventions. For example, as noted above, anxiety and depression often require cognitive-behavioral therapy, as well as medications that are not ADHD medications per se. And learning disorders do not respond directly to the behavioral contingencies and medications that are typically the treatment of choice for ADHD. In such cases, direct academic remediation is in order.

So, if ADHD is not "all that there is," it's essential to get treatment for your daughter's related behavior and emotional patterns.

Putting It All Together

Overall, evaluating a girl (or boy) for ADHD is not something that should be taken lightly or done quickly. As I've taken pains to elaborate in this chapter, the core procedures are careful observations of behaviors, cognitive performance, and emotional responses within the home, school, and peer environments. Using rating scales/questionnaires from parents and teachers, detailed interviews with the family, a medical exam to rule out other conditions, and sometimes a variety of one-on-one tests, the clinician tries to "build a case" for diagnosing the consistent and impairing inconsistencies in performance that are the hallmark of ADHD. At the same time, the evaluator must be aware of and assess for the variety of additional conditions that frequently accompany (or can mask as) ADHD, as these disorders nearly always require additional treatment strategies. And lest we forget, assessment of strengths is also a must.

It's rare, both in my experience and large amounts of research, that a girl reveals a classic pattern of disorganization, forgetfulness, trouble with impulse control, and substandard school performance without additional anxiety, depression, oppositionality, posttraumatic reactions, or specific learning disorders. When there are no comorbid disorders, evidence-based treatments for ADHD often work quickly and effectively. But in the real world, such factors as comorbid diagnoses, family stress, overcrowded classrooms, and early trauma can greatly complicate the diagnosis and treatment plan.

Finally, you will undoubtedly have a range of reactions and responses to the clinician's feedback that your daughter indeed has ADHD, if that's the result of the evaluation. You may be incredulous, initially denying that a child of yours meets criteria for this condition. Or you may grieve the "typical" daughter you thought you were raising. Or you may actually be relieved that there's finally a diagnosis—which might help you transcend a lot of the guilt and shame you've been experiencing with respect to ongoing family struggles. Through reading this book, as well as examining the Resources after the last chapter, you are coming to realize that ADHD in girls brings on a number of serious life issues and impairments, but it also provides the opportunity to reevaluate your daughter and your relationship with her, toward the end of forging the kinds of treatment planning that are the main subject of the second half of this book. Overall, in this chapter I reiterated the concepts from Chapter 1 of forging a *radical acceptance* of your daughter, in light of the ADHD she is experiencing, along with a *radical commitment* to make key changes in your home life and secure the best services possible for her and your family.

In the end, the diagnostic evaluation, along with the feedback and the many inevitable reactions you may experience, does not mean that the future is bleak for your daughter. As you'll see in the next chapter—and, in fact, in the rest of the book—the outlook for a girl with ADHD can be bright, with your love, commitment, and attention and an emphasis on all of her strengths and talents. Still, the commitment is often substantial.

THREE

What Is the Outlook
for Girls with ADHD?

If you read Chapters 1 and 2, you should be getting a foundational understanding of ADHD and forming an idea of whether your daughter has the disorder. But what does this mean for her future? My goal for this chapter is to take you beyond your daughter's childhood—and even her adolescence—into what's known about her potential longer-term future.

Unfortunately, the scientific and clinical communities still do not know enough about this topic to provide a full set of authoritative answers. Why? Well, as you may recall from Chapter 1, the longstanding male bias in research and clinical practice related to ADHD has left us with very little research evidence on the long-term outcomes for girls with ADHD. By definition, follow-up research—termed *longitudinal* by researchers in this area, with the goal of discovering adult outcomes—requires many years between childhood and adulthood. Because, with rare exceptions, girls were believed not to qualify for an ADHD diagnosis until the 1990s, there just aren't many data available with respect to adult follow-up. One of the reasons I chose to write this book is that my own research team at the University of California (UC), Berkeley has worked with the largest study in existence of girls with ADHD, carefully diagnosed prior to adolescence. We have followed them into their 20s (and in the current wave of data collection, into their 30s). As a result, I'll be sharing with you some of the most important findings from this, and other, longitudinal research on this essential area.

But before diving into the findings, I'd like to give you a deeper sense of what the transitions into adolescence and then adulthood look like for girls in general, beyond those with ADHD. I became interested in this topic in large part because of our team's follow-up studies, which have involved not only girls (and boys) with ADHD but comparison groups of typically developing children. Witnessing the life-course trajectories of our typically developing comparison girls awakened me to the issues that all girls experience as they mature. As a result, I've done a lot of reading and thinking about the larger social, cultural, and biological issues related to girls' transitions into adolescence and beyond. There isn't room here for a full, yearlong seminar on this topic, but I hope that my introduction can give you some real food for thought in your effort to understand the potential for particularly serious long-term outcomes of girls who experience challenges like ADHD. Let's begin with adolescence.

Adolescence in Girls

How do we define *adolescence?* In developmental terms, we usually define this period by when it begins and ends, but surprisingly, those shifts are not that easy to pin down.

When Does Adolescence Begin?

The "teens" begin at 13, as evidenced by the last syllable of the numbers (and years of age) from 13 to 19. A biological definition of adolescence would involve the body's maturation into adult forms and functions, which allow sexual reproduction, a process called *puberty.* But puberty is not all or none. Rather, it is a process that takes place over years. For girls, the formal onset of puberty is often defined as the age of the first menstrual period, termed *menarche.* The average age of menarche was between 14 and 15 in the late 19th century, but it has dipped to 12 or so at present. For certain racial groups, like Black girls, the average age is even earlier, around 11. Note that boys have also shown a decrease in their age of sexual maturation, but they remain, on average, a year or more later than girls. Factors like better overall nutrition (and hormone content in current diets), a higher percentage of girls who are overweight, and surrounding chemicals in the environment could all be playing a role. Whatever the causes, adolescence, defined biologically, is beginning ever earlier in our current world.

An early transition into physical maturity is not usually much of a problem for boys; it may actually confer some advantages (for example, not being a victim of bullying). Yet early menarche and physical development for girls can predict a number of negative outcomes. Especially when combined with other risk factors, they can put girls in the path of predatory males and propel a cycle of low academic engagement, substance use, and more.

When Does Adolescence End?

On the other side, how do we know when adolescence ends? Here, the definition is more social and cultural than strictly biological. That is, if we are referring to the age at which individuals attain economic independence and start their own families, this milestone is reached far later in development than at other times in human history—often into one's 20s or beyond. Think of the years of education and training that are mandatory for so many jobs these days, or the kinds of resources and life skills needed to launch a family.

The New Adolescence: Emerging Adulthood

The bottom line is that puberty and adolescence are beginning ever earlier in the current world, especially for girls, and that adolescence is stretching well beyond age 18 or 19 for many if not most young people. In fact, psychologists have begun calling the age range from around 18 or 19 through the mid- or late 20s *emerging adulthood,* signaling the prolonged period before one achieves full adult status. This "gap" between physical maturity and emotional and financial independence places huge strain on teens, particularly girls.

Intriguingly, with the advent of brain imaging (see Chapter 2), scientists now know far more than before about the brain's development from childhood through adulthood. From a set of well-publicized findings that initially appeared in neuroscience research about 20 years ago, a crucial discovery has been that full brain maturation for youth occurs particularly slowly for the frontal lobes, especially the prefrontal cortex (the outermost layer of the brain located just behind the forehead). This is a neural region that is highly interconnected with other brain areas; it is deeply involved in planning, inhibiting responses, and the other executive functions that were noted in Chapter 2. In fact, this area of the brain does not attain its full adult maturity until the mid-20s, on average, for females—and several years later for males. Little wonder that adolescence is a time of peak physical and cognitive strength but also a time of high risk for accidents, drug use, and other consequences of impulsive behavior—given that the frontal areas of the brain are not fully equipped to put the brakes on the surge for independence that characterizes the teen years. In short, even at a biological level, "adolescence" certainly does not suddenly end at 18 or 19.

At a 30,000-foot level, the first 10 years of life are a high-risk period for a number of boys to experience autism, ADHD, movement disorders, and early-onset conduct problems—at rates above those found in girls (see Chapter 1). Boys are generally slower to mature than girls, putting them at risk for many neurodevelopmental conditions. But the second 10 years of life, comprising the preteen and teen years, witness greatly heightened risk for girls in terms of depression, anxiety, self-harm (suicidal behavior, as well as cutting and other forms of nonsuicidal self-injury, or NSSI), eating-related symptoms—and even increases in antisocial behavior.

And disturbingly, this heightened risk in adolescence for girls has actually *grown* in the past 25 years. That is, girls are more likely than ever to experience anxiety and depression and binge eating. Teen girls' rates of aggressive behavior have also increased over the past several decades, whereas boys' rates have gone down. In particular, self-harm and suicidal behavior—which combine "internalizing" (as in depression) and "externalizing" (aggression, but directed toward the self)—have risen precipitously for girls in recent years.

The question is why. It's almost impossible to believe that the surges in such problems for girls result from sudden changes in underlying genetic vulnerability (evolutionary trends take many generations to emerge). Something toxic at a *cultural* level could well be driving these trends.

> *To fully understand the impact of ADHD on girls, you first have to understand the impact of society's messages on all girls.*

I wrote a book on this very issue in 2009, called *The Triple Bind: Saving our Teenage Girls from Today's Pressures.* My belief is that forces in society increasingly drive girls into serious psychological consequences—especially girls who already have underlying vulnerabilities, like ADHD. The headlines of this perspective are that society expects the following:

1. Girls must continue to be compliant and nurturing, the traits expected of females throughout history.

2. They often outperform boys academically and athletically, because we have finally given girls core opportunities, adding a conflicting pressure.

3. They must do both of the above in a hypersexualized and effortless manner.

Yet pulling off this *triple bind* is both physically and psychologically impossible. Thus, teen girls are placed in an untenable situation, in which they cannot (no one can!) pull off this combination of empathy, competitiveness, and effortless sexuality. When they inevitably fail in this regard, decreases in self-image and increases in destructive behavior are predictable.

You can read about the implications of the triple bind for all adolescent girls in more detail in the box on pages 69–72. But what is important for this book is how the triple bind affects a girl entering her teen years who has already experienced the kinds of dysregulated attention, disorganization, lack of self-control, and poor impulse control characteristic of ADHD since childhood. Here, the impossible pressures of the triple bind are greatly magnified.

In *The Triple Bind* I described an admittedly unethical thought experiment: What if researchers got a bunch of teen girls together in a sealed room for days or weeks and piped in tobacco smoke? Just about everyone would get red eyes, develop a cough, and experience intense physical distress. Some might have to deal with lasting effects. Yet those with early asthma, a genetic vulnerability to lung cancer, or other vulnerabilities would be the ones with the most dire long-term consequences.

Replace the physical poison (tobacco smoke) with the cultural "toxin" of the triple bind, replete with its impossible expectations. It wouldn't be piped into an enclosed room—because it's in the everyday environments girls experience, all the time. It would be hard to imagine that any girl could escape some level of conflict and distress. But those with the underlying symptoms of ADHD—the risk that is strongly related to genes (see Chapter 4)—would be prone to show accelerated and deeper risk for later impairment and suffering.

Many questions remain. Does the triple bind exist only in Westernized countries? What's the "right" kind of academic pressure for society to place on youth in this ever-escalating world of digital and verbal literacy? Are boys vulnerable to increasing pressures as well? As for this last question, many contend that male culture and male development are becoming increasingly devalued these days, leaving boys vulnerable to a low sense of self-worth. Still, teen boys have real space for performance-based success without the additional expectations of being completely caring and nurturing and looking particularly "hot." In fact, if an academically or athletically successful adolescent guy also happens also to be particularly kind and caring, we often think (or say out loud): How remarkable! Yet if a successful girl has her accomplishments come at the expense of complete empathy, we'd wonder what's wrong with her or her family.

With this information at hand, let's consider research on what transpires for girls with ADHD over the long haul. I'll be the first to admit that some of the findings below are startling, in terms of how ADHD can predispose girls to some truly negative outcomes. But please view the averages considered in the next section in light of the potential for strength and thriving as girls with ADHD mature. In fact, as I emphasize in the second half of the book, perhaps the most important task ahead of you is to seek out and promote your daughter's intrinsic interests and strengths. Doing so not only provides needed rewards for the behavioral programs you'll be establishing for her but also points the way toward successes as she matures. Finally, when I point out the factors that help to explain long-term impairments, you'll see that this analysis can lead to avenues for help.

Long-Term Outcomes for Girls with ADHD: What Do We Know?

Clinical researchers have been following up boys (or almost exclusively boys) with ADHD for over half a century. In broad strokes, these scientists have found that boys diagnosed with ADHD (or earlier labels, in the oldest research):

- Experience curtailed academic achievement scores and lower academic attainment (like postsecondary degrees) than do those in comparison groups
- Are far more likely than their peers to demonstrate aggressive and delinquent behavior as well as chronic antisocial behavior in adulthood
- Have elevated rates of alcohol and nicotine use, along with rates of usage of illicit substances

The evidence is less consistent for anxiety, depression, and other "internalizing" conditions, although most studies reveal that heightened risk does exist in boys.

For girls, however, only two sizable follow-up studies exist: (1) the Massachusetts General Hospital (MGH) sample, featuring 140 carefully diagnosed girls with ADHD ages 6–17 years at the study's onset, plus a nearly equal-sized comparison group, and (2) the Berkeley Girls with ADHD Longitudinal Study (BGALS), noted at the beginning of this chapter, also featuring 140 girls with ADHD ages 6–12 years at "baseline," along with 88 matched comparison girls.

The MGH study revealed that, into late adolescence and early adulthood, girls originally diagnosed with ADHD:

- Demonstrated rates of antisocial, mood, anxiety, developmental, addictive, and eating disorders substantially higher than those for the comparison girls (though the aggressive and antisocial behavior patterns had a later onset than for boys)

- Had higher rates of mood and anxiety disorders than boys with ADHD, although the girls with ADHD showed lower rates of adult antisocial behaviors than the boys did

- Revealed compromised executive functions

Although the MGH sample was predominantly White and did not represent impoverished girls, the findings clearly showed that ADHD in girls, on average, yields problems that persist for over 10 years.

The box on pages 72–75 describes our BGALS sample in some detail, along with key findings as the girls matured beyond adolescence. This sample is ethnically and racially diverse, and it includes girls from families of a wide range of income levels. By the age ranges of the early 20s and then the mid- to late 20s, several key findings from the BGALS became apparent:

> *Research findings show that ADHD creates problems that endure in girls for at least a decade, on average.*

- Girls with ADHD often-showed substantial academic, social, cognitive, and behavioral problems, well beyond those of the comparison group.

- The most notable impairments were found in the areas of depression, self-harm, intimate relationships (for example, experiences of partner violence and unplanned pregnancy), and postsecondary educational and job-related functioning.

- These impairments were often linked with "taking it out on themselves" via self-harm, or being victimized, in sometimes devastating ways.

Some girls, however, have thrived. And, as with outcomes in adult life for almost everyone, for the majority there was a mixed picture of strengths and weaknesses. The aim for the rest of the chapters in this book is to aid you in helping your daughter along the road to thriving.

What We Learned about Self-Harm in Girls with ADHD

The most striking findings related to girls' ultrahigh risk for NSSI and suicidal behavior. Frankly, my research team and I were stunned when we learned of these results over a decade ago. It was clear that many girls with ADHD, once entering late adolescence and adulthood, had problems that did not fade away—and this outcome too often revealed considerable dissatisfaction with their lives. Their issues may not have been as overtly visible as acting-out behavior, delinquency, or florid substance abuse, more typically found in boys with ADHD. But they were all too real to the young women who experienced them, as well as their families. The core question, though, is "Why do they occur?"

> The self-harm that is all too common in girls with ADHD may be far less visible to others than the acting out of boys, but it can easily be as devastating.

What Factors Increase the Risk of Self-Harm?

First, my research team scoured the many measures we collected when the BGALS participants were girls, in order to discover which behaviors and processes predicted self-destructive behaviors by emerging adulthood or beyond. Here's what we found:

- High levels of impulsivity, as indicated from the finding that it was primarily the girls with childhood ADHD–Combined who had the highest risk
- High levels of inattention—intriguingly, this also emerged as a predictor of later suicide attempts, when we examined inattention as a continuum of behavior rather than just a "presentation" of ADHD
- Low self-esteem (sometimes called *poor self-concept*)

- Poor executive functions—especially related to planning and general self-control

- Negative interactions with dads, even beyond negative interactions with moms; and high levels of parenting stress in the primary caregiver, most often the mom (I will have much more to say about family functioning and family interactions in Chapter 5)

- Noncompliant/aggressive behaviors (these were particularly strong predictors of NSSI)

- Anxious and depressed behavior patterns (especially regarding suicidality)

- Adverse experiences in childhood, including mental illness in family members, maltreatment, separation/divorce, and more

The bottom line is that for girls, ADHD in childhood comes with a range of added factors that can leave them, by adolescence and adulthood, with the sense that negative emotions are intolerable or that, in fact, life is not worth living—predicting NSSI or suicidal behavior. Notably, the strongest predictors of self-harm were often *combinations* of childhood risk factors. For example, 80% of participants with adolescent or young-adult NSSI had childhood aggressive and depressive scores in the clinical range *along with* poor childhood executive functioning.

> *The childhood experience of ADHD can leave teen girls and adult women believing that distressing emotions are unbearable—with a need to express pain in harmful ways—and even that life may not be worth living.*

> *The experience of girls with ADHD dispels the notion that only disruptive, impulsive childhood behavior patterns—more typical of boys—lead to later problems.*

We also found extraordinarily high rates of unplanned pregnancy in the BGALS sample. Here, it turned out that both childhood inattention and childhood impulsivity played a predictive role. In fact, for a range of other outcomes, in both boys and girls with ADHD, it's not just the more visible impulsive and hyperactive behaviors but also inattentive/disorganized behavior patterns in childhood that are potent precursors of substance use, driving accidents, and low academic achievement.

How Do Risks Predict Outcomes?

The design of the BGALS follow-up assessments has allowed us to examine not only factors and variables in childhood that predict real impairment later on but also processes during adolescence that help us understand how the risks eventuate in difficult outcomes. In the language of psychology, variables that occur in the time period between a *risk factor* (like ADHD) and an *outcome* (like engagement in self-harm or unplanned pregnancy) are called *mediators*—that is, intermediate processes that help to explain how the initial risk yields the later-life problem. In fact, we have found important explanatory factors during adolescence that help us understand how such negative outcomes may have arisen.

> *The more we learn about what turns a risk factor into a negative outcome, the more we can prevent adolescent and adult problems from plaguing girls with ADHD.*

Even more important, this information could be of real relevance in *preventing* some of the difficult outcomes experienced by girls with ADHD:

1. **In the area of NSSI, the following adolescent factors come into play:**
   - Aggressive behavior as reported by parents and teachers
   - Poor ability to inhibit impulsive actions
   - The experience of being victimized by peers, either physically or verbally

2. **Different factors helped to explain attempted suicide:**
   - High levels of anxiety and depression, reported by participants and caregivers
   - The experience of exclusion from peer groups (in other words, low social acceptance from agemates)
   - Physical abuse, sexual abuse, or neglect in either childhood or

adolescence (technically, note that depending on the girl's age at the time, this could be considered as either a predictor or a mediator)

3. **Two factors seemed to explain the elevated risk for unplanned pregnancy:**

   - Low academic performance in early to mid-adolescence
   - Risky sexual behavior in later adolescence

For unplanned pregnancy, we uncovered a kind of "chain reaction," whereby childhood ADHD, when followed by low academic performance in middle school and early high school—which then predicted engaging in high-risk sexual behavior—was the pathway most strongly linked to unplanned pregnancy. Furthermore, the key adolescent factor that protected against the experience of intimate partner violence was also high levels of academic achievement.

> *High academic achievement is a key protective factor against intimate partner violence for girls with ADHD.*

As I address in the following section, these factors can help us understand and intervene, when our goal is to curtail some of the most difficult outcomes faced by girls with ADHD on their developmental paths. Key points to remember:

- Both inattention and hyperactive-impulsive behavior in childhood and adolescence predict negative outcomes in later life for girls with ADHD. It's not just the most noticeable and disruptive behaviors that count!

- Both acting-out/aggressive behaviors and depression contribute to later difficulties as well.

- Experiences at home (early adverse experiences, severe mistreatment, parenting stress, and negative parent–child interchanges—particularly with fathers) are also crucial.

- Low academic achievement (sometimes accompanied by low executive functioning) is a key link between childhood ADHD and several later impairments for girls. Keeping your daughter engaged in school, which may often require additional supports, is vital.

- Difficulties with peer interactions, including both victimization by and frank rejection from agemates, are explanatory. As well, when academic failure is occurring, your daughter may become attracted to peers interested in quick rewards—like sexual contact and drug use.

 • Low self-esteem, which is synonymous with a poor sense of self-worth, is critical. I'll have more to say about enhancing self-worth in the next section.

What Can You Do to Promote Resilience and Thriving?

You may be reacting to the findings above with the same dismay that my team and I did when we started to look at our results. There is no denying that ADHD can lead to some particularly troublesome outcomes for girls. Even more, a number of studies of women with ADHD from around the world confirm that high rates of self-harm, problems in the workplace, and early pregnancy/childbirth are significant outcomes. Still, we've found that a considerable number of BGALS participants who struggled with self-harm in their adolescence and early adulthood stopped engaging in such behaviors as they matured. As well, many who had difficulties in finding the right kinds of schooling or with attempts toward independence have succeeded, albeit sometimes after many tries. *In other words, it's never too late.* The story of one young woman's journey to success in the box on pages 75–77 is an inspiring example.

> *Research shows that as they mature, many girls with ADHD leave behind self-harm, academic difficulties, and struggles to reach independence—with good supports in place.*

Importantly, the information above provides clear clues as to the kinds of practices that may help to prevent some of the worst outcomes described in the preceding pages. Chapters 6 through 9 provide specific focus on evidence-based treatments for ADHD—including several forms of behavioral and cognitive-behavioral interventions as well as medications, for both girls and teens. But this is a good time to learn how to maintain your, your family's, and your daughter's motivation for change, no matter how old she may be.

Staying Engaged

By the early teen and teen years, many girls—and particularly those with ADHD—give off the vibe that they are done with their families, wanting nothing to do with you, their parent. At the same time, although you may not realize it, most of them still are desperately seeking parental outreach. Given shame over failure experiences, a history of negative family interactions, and/or challenges with friendships, the façade is often one of disgruntlement and distance.

A true challenge is staying positive and encouraging, amid the seemingly constant battles (and amid the stress you are likely to experience) in your parenting role. Please: seek openings despite the stonewalling. That is, let your daughter know that you are "there" and ready to talk when she is. Try to relish what she does well despite the conflict and arguments (much more on promoting strengths comes in the latter half of this book). Continue to be patient when your patience seems gone. All of this falls under the umbrella of radical acceptance. In many instances, your perseverance and underlying faith in your daughter can lead to welcome contact, sometimes when you least expect it. It can also help her stay involved in treatment—especially if the family is similarly engaged in active intervention, showing her that everyone is working, both separately and together.

Encouraging School Engagement

As emphasized above, poor academic performance is a potent factor on the path from early ADHD to later unplanned pregnancies, intimate partner violence, and a range of additional problems. Beyond symptom management, it makes good sense to do whatever you can to keep your daughter with ADHD identified with and thriving in her academic work, especially during the transitions to middle school and high school.

How? Perhaps by searching for the right school if the present one just isn't working. Or gaining accommodations (or additional accommodations) in the current school. Or by securing tutoring—or providing extra incentives for homework completion (see Chapter 7 for more on education). Medication, if at the right dosage, can facilitate attention and increase academic performance, as can contracts related to a behavioral program. (More on medication and behavioral programs can be found in Chapter 6.) Staying in touch with the teachers who relate well to your daughter and see her strengths is crucial, as is outreach toward the teachers with whom your daughter is having the greatest difficulties.

Self-Esteem

Self-esteem is interesting: If too high, the individual may feel entitled and not terribly motivated to change. If too low, the individual may be paralyzed by deficient motivation, helplessness, and even shame. A sense of self-worth that's relatively stable (not rising or falling each day on the tides of external feedback)—and that's positive, but not overly so—may be the ideal.

Girls with ADHD tend to have low-esteem. As I've shown, such low self-regard, especially when paired with other risk factors, can increase the likelihood of serious outcomes such as self-harm.

But wait: I am not implying that you should overzealously praise your daughter (or anyone else!) in an attempt to prop up an overly (and falsely) inflated self-image. Self-esteem is not something to be promoted at all costs. Instead, it will rise naturally with family support, gradual successes, and a growing sense of true interests and goals, rather than via the "false self" and false ideals that the triple bind too often promotes. We clearly want to avoid an overly positive sense of self-esteem that may not be grounded in reality.

Make sure your daughter knows you're there for her at every step, and encourage her—with needed treatment, supports, and accommodations—to take steps in a world that seems too often to discourage her. In other words, in a nutshell, embrace radical commitment. Stable, generally positive self-esteem can be a bastion of safety in an unpredictable world, too often filled with failure experiences if you have serious ADHD.

Friendships and Peer Relationships

You may well feel that you have little control over whom your daughter chooses as friends or who chooses her. Starting in childhood, helping with play-dates can be a good thing, especially when she is lacking in social skills and may need encouragement. During the tricky preadolescent and adolescent years, you have less control over peer contacts. Keep in mind, though, that even one positive friendship can provide a counterbalance when a girl seems to be lacking in popularity and overall peer support. As long as you don't come across as overly controlling or directive, you can also talk with your daughter about the qualities she admires in friends, to assist her with good decision making.

As any child matures, parents need to strike a balance between gradually reducing control and limits while still providing the kinds of monitoring to prevent their offspring from hanging out with the wrong crowd. Of course, this is easier said than done when your daughter tends to push aside limits of any kind that you try to set. When such is the case, family interventions are often indicated.

Above All: Competence and Engagement

Perhaps the strongest advice I can give is to help your daughter find areas of competence and joyful engagement—and give her as many chances as possible to participate in such activities. These may not be in traditional areas of academic or athletic accomplishment. In fact, discovering her interests is an intriguing challenge. As you open up communication, make a point of becoming interested in and supportive of her proclivities and gently guide her preferred directions. In the process, you may find talents and interests that you weren't even sure she had. Overall, the classic research on promoting well-being strongly suggests two key protective factors: (1) positive, healthy relationships (in or outside the home) and (2) promoting strengths. Relatives, coaches, mentors, community leaders, favorite teachers—all may be able to help play such roles.

Overall, I urge you to read the boxes at the end of the chapter. You'll get more information regarding pathways that girls with ADHD have taken between their earliest years and later-life outcomes, from the two existing major research studies and from an individual who has traveled that path. I hope that you, as do I, believe that there is a lot to learn.

At this point, we're ready to tackle what causes ADHD, along with more information about the roles that families and family interactions play in the course of ADHD over development.

The "Triple Bind"

In *The Triple Bind*, I wrote about a potential explanation for the rising rates of serious mental health problems in teenage girls. Here's a synopsis.

First, in our modern world, the overwhelming tendency still exists to expect girls, as they develop, to be empathic, sensitive, nurturing, and caregiving. Yes, boys and men have a broader range of possibilities than previously with respect to showing feelings, assisting with child rearing, and providing support to others. Still, the predominant expectation is that females should carry the day in these domains.

Second, however, over the last generation-plus, political and social movements, along with general cultural trends in many nations and societies, have pushed for expanded rights and opportunities for girls and women. In the United States, for example, the drive toward equal opportunities for females in education, athletics, and employment has been palpable. Although complete equality is far from a reality, real progress has occurred. Think, for example, of Title IX, first enacted in 1972, which prohibits discrimination on the basis of sex for any education program that receives federal assistance. Title IX applies largely but not exclusively to athletics and has opened up a former male bastion to girls and women. At the same time, the Women's Movement and other forms of political activism have served to expand a number of additional opportunities to females.

As a result, college, graduate school, and professional education have opened up admissions for women, with many pervasively held stereotypes broken (for example, that girls and women are "naturally" inferior to men in sciences and math). Although some fields are slower to change than others, at present girls perform equivalently to boys in high-school math. Admissions to 4-year colleges and universities have favored women over men for more than 40 years, with the proportion growing over time. Admissions to medical and law schools favor females over males as well, by a slight margin, compared to men-only policies several generations ago.

The bottom line is that, in light of more equal opportunities, girls now outcompete boys academically in many areas of study—and female athletes are now revered in many sports. Yet how do you, as a girl, cross the finish line first, or obtain that prestigious scholarship, when you're also judged by how nurturing you are to others? It's difficult indeed to win the race while being tempted to help the other girl who has staggered or fallen near the finish line. In short, over the past half-century, and at an ever-increasing rate, girls experience a real conflict between the first two "prongs" of the triple bind— that is, caregiving versus competing. And let's remember that the increased opportunities for girls and women don't often come with commensurate compensation, making things truly confusing for females.

Third, the last prong of the triple bind is less overt but still real. Specifically, you're not performing the juggling act between being empathic and competitive as a female should unless you (1) do so effortlessly ("don't let them see you sweat") and (2) look "hot" (that is, sexualized) as you try. In other words, if you show your struggle and don't maintain an ultrafeminine, sexualized appearance, you really haven't succeeded in terms of the feminine ideal.

The Triple Bind and related research have provided substantial evidence to bolster these perspectives. The crucial point is that it is simply impossible, physically and psychologically, to negotiate all three aspects of the triple bind. Yet if, as a teenage girl, you have "bought" and internalized the belief that you simply have to pull it off, the consequences can be devastating. For one thing, you would tend to internalize the pressures and inherent conflict—blaming yourself if you can't do the impossible. In fact, *internalizing* is the psychological term for anxiety, depression, symptoms of eating disorders, and many aspects of self-destructive behavior. Internalization as a process clearly predicts internalizing (depressed, anxious) disorders. Given the continuing surge in mental health issues for girls, the arguments I presented over a decade ago in support of the noxious consequences of the triple bind are even stronger today than they were then.

From a different angle, we have come to realize just how essential sleep is for physical and emotional well-being. But if you're a teenage girl caught up in the triple bind, how is there room for more than a few hours of sleep each night (including the pressures of social media to stay connected with peers, online, on a nearly 24/7 schedule)? When one is sleep-deprived, beyond physical exhaustion, negative emotions predominate over positive emotions, further exacerbating the development of internalizing conditions.

Furthermore, the goal of adolescence is, in many ways, to work on developing a true sense of self. Doing so requires an honest appraisal of strengths, weaknesses, and coping resources. But the triple bind is all about doing impossible things to reach an unattainable goal. As a result, unrealistic expectations and self-imposed pressure are prone to plague far too many girls even after their teen years.

Finally, there's a psychological term called *learned helplessness*. It was coined over 50 years ago in application to experimental animals who were given uncontrollable electric shocks when harnessed into stalls. Even when the bars of the stall were removed, those that had received uncontrollable shocks essentially just stood there when the shocks stopped. They had apparently been conditioned that no matter what they did when receiving the shocks, it didn't matter. How many teenage girls exposed to the uncontrollable and relentless barrage of the triple bind remain in the thrall of those expectations even if the messages somehow stop? The answer, I fear, is,

"Too many." Add to those messages and expectations an ongoing experience of ADHD-linked difficulties, and the results can too often be devastating.

The Berkeley Girls with ADHD Longitudinal Study (BGALS)

During the early 1990s, I became convinced that the party line—namely, girls either don't experience ADHD or do so quite rarely—was misguided. I had been working almost exclusively with boys diagnosed with ADHD since the time of my doctoral dissertation some years earlier but never gathered enough girls with ADHD to create a viable study. So, I wrote a research grant to the National Institute of Mental Health (NIMH) asking for funds to put in place, in an all-girl milieu, the summer camp methodology I'd been using for many years with boys. In brief, children with ADHD participated together with typically developing kids in an enrichment program allowing for plentiful observations of behavior in real-world contexts. On my second attempt at a long grant application, the reviewers and NIMH agreed that this was a high-priority area, and funds arrived.

Still, while giving talks to school districts, sending fliers to Bay Area pediatricians, and advertising the program in other ways, a nagging question lingered: What if there actually weren't enough girls out there to conduct the study? This question received a quick answer in the early spring of 1997, a few months before the start of the first of the three summer enrichment programs: The day we opened our new telephone line, the phone nearly rang off the hook.

Across the next three years, with over 1,000 inquiries, we carefully screened parents and their daughters via an intensive set of calls, rating scales, interviews, and tests, using the kinds of evidence-based assessment procedures described in Chapter 2 but including even more detail. We also videotaped girls and their parents interacting with each other to get a sense of family dynamics. In the end, across 1997, 1998, and 1999, we diagnosed 140 girls, ages 6–12 years, with either ADHD–Combined or ADHD–Inattentive. We also selected 88 comparison girls without ADHD in the same age range, from the same communities and the same diverse racial and ethnic groups, to attend one of our three all-girl research summer programs. After the intensive initial assessments, we studied the girls as they participated alongside one another, with neither participants nor staff aware of who was in which particular diagnostic group.

The programs provided an enriching set of classroom, art, drama, and playground/athletic experiences. Counselors and teachers provided daily ratings on "narrow" questionnaires, and trained college students made precise observations of behavior patterns. Each week, the girls privately rated one another, to ascertain measures of peer acceptance and peer rejection. We also administered a host of one-on-one measures of emotions, behaviors, and attitudes.

It would take far too long to describe the many findings. In short, we found that the girls with ADHD had worse performance in reading and math, poorer executive functioning, higher rates of being disliked by their peers (and friendships marked by considerable conflict), more reactive emotional behaviors, lower self-esteem, greater levels of parental stress, and higher rates of both anxiety/depression and oppositional/aggressive behavior than the comparison girls did.

Importantly, in findings that came as a surprise, we found that girls with the inattentive presentation of ADHD (that is, with high levels of inattention or disorganization but not hyperactivity or impulsivity) and girls with the combined form (that is, with high levels of both symptom types) were almost indistinguishable with respect to just about all of the impairments we measured. The only exceptions were that girls with ADHD–Combined showed higher levels of aggressive behavior patterns during the programs—and were more likely to be shunned by their peers. Overall, girls with "pure" inattention had real-world impairments comparable to those with inattention plus impulsivity.

Yet our key goal was to follow the participants well past the summer programs in childhood (Wave 1). Through a series of additional grants, we reevaluated the participants during early adolescence (Wave 2, average age of 14–15), late adolescence/emerging adulthood (Wave 3, average age of 19–20), and the beginning of adulthood (Wave 4, average age of 25–26). Through diligent efforts, we were able to follow up between 92% and 95% of our participants across the waves. Because an acronym can be a good thing, the study became known as the Berkeley Girls with ADHD Longitudinal Study (BGALS).

At each wave, we assessed a wide range of outcomes, using many of the same measures administered at Wave 1. We also added assessments of issues that become salient in adolescence and adulthood. These included such areas as delinquency, drug use, close relationships, and self-harm. The latter area involves both NSSI (involving cutting and other forms of self-damage without the intent to die) and attempted suicide (actions taken with the intent of ending one's life). With respect to NSSI, it may be hard to imagine that one would cut or burn oneself—but such actions are escalating rapidly in teens, especially girls.

Revealing that ADHD is not a transitory problem for females, the majority of the girls diagnosed at Wave 1 continued to meet criteria for ADHD at later waves. Even when symptom counts had receded by adulthood, however, key problems and impairments tended to persist. Across every domain of impairment we evaluated, the girls with ADHD, on average, showed greater dysfunction. Their adult performance in math was particularly low—nearly half met criteria for a learning disorder in mathematics. And their deficient executive functioning in childhood persisted into adulthood. Crucially, not only childhood impulsivity but also childhood inattention accounted for continuing impairment in most outcomes. Just because ADHD may not be as visible or annoying in girls with the inattentive form does *not* mean that things will automatically "clear up" in adolescence and beyond.

Clinically important differences from the findings of male follow-up studies emerged. For one thing, the BGALS participants with childhood ADHD did not show the same levels of delinquent behavior as do most male samples. Even more, except for tobacco use, the BGALS girls with ADHD did not reveal the same kinds of overall substance abuse patterns as have most male samples. Instead, the realms of internalizing behavior patterns (specifically depression and anxiety), self-harm, close relationships, and postsecondary education/job performance stood out.

A capsule summary: Girls with ADHD showed higher rates of later depression than did the comparisons, at rates above those in most male follow-up studies. Furthermore, by adolescence and early adulthood, they also disclosed alarmingly high rates of self-harm. Let me elaborate.

NSSI ranges from cuticle-picking and mild hair-pulling to serious acts of cutting one's skin, burning oneself, or banging one's head against hard objects. A core idea is that when teens experience really difficult and toxic emotions, with no apparent solution, they might engage in NSSI as a means of experiencing physical pain, which temporarily (but only temporarily) alleviates the deeper emotional distress. A vicious cycle can often ensue, with escalating levels of self-injury. I should note that a history of NSSI can itself be a risk factor for eventual suicidal behavior.

We found that by an average age of 20, 19% of the comparison sample was engaging in moderate to severe NSSI, versus 29% of the those with childhood ADHD–Inattentive and fully 51% of those with ADHD–Combined. In terms of attempted suicide, the rates were 6% for the comparisons, 8% for ADHD–Inattentive, and 22.4% for those with ADHD–Combined. (In case you're wondering, the comparison-group NSSI rate of 19% and attempted suicide rate of 6% are squarely within national averages. In other words, our California sample does not appear to be an outlier.) These percentages climbed slightly by Wave 4 (average age of 26 years), although many girls had desisted from self-harm by then. Thus, ADHD in girls, particularly when marked by both inattention and substantial impulsivity, is a clear risk factor for self-harm—even more so than in boys with ADHD.

Also salient were the domains of intimate partner violence (our participants with ADHD had received high amounts) and unplanned pregnancy. In fact, by Wave 4, 43% of the ADHD sample had experienced at least one unplanned pregnancy, in contrast to 11% of the comparisons—a whopping difference. In addition, although the vast majority of BGALS participants with ADHD ended up graduating from high school, their postsecondary educational experiences were hugely variable and quite often less than successful. As well, we found greater levels of job-related problems than in the comparison women.

It's one thing to document that, on average, girls with ADHD continue to experience key problems beyond their preadolescent years, particularly and tragically in areas that involve self-harm. More important, however, is the attempt to explain (1) the kinds of childhood factors and adolescent processes that underlie such long-term impairments and (2) the processes that predict successes in many girls with ADHD.

What If You Don't Get Diagnosed with ADHD Until Graduate School?

Sara Chung, PhD, a brilliant clinical psychologist, recently received her doctorate from UC Berkeley. Her narrative conveys how difficult it can be to struggle for years with the shame and stigma accompanying severe but undiagnosed inattention—and how an accurate diagnosis and responsive treatment can be welcome at any time. This is her story, in her own words, which she wrote in an attempt to share an important personal narrative and to overcome stigma.

• • •

My parents are non-English-speaking immigrants from China who have faced the stresses of acculturation and financial instability for four decades in the United States. Like many second-generation children, I struggled to learn English, navigate the American educational system, and make friends with other American children with limited support from my parents. By the end of elementary school, my parents could no longer understand my academic demands nor the implications of teachers' comments that I was inattentive.

It was not until I was diagnosed with ADHD–Inattentive at the age of 31—and in the fourth year of an intensive PhD program—that I began to understand just how deeply my untreated attentional challenges had affected my well-being, social interactions, goals and pursuits, and identity.

Since childhood, my sense of self was predominantly based on being an imposter. At school, I was seen as a bright student whose test scores placed me in the Gifted and Talented Education program. I turned in flawless assignments and earned top marks. What I hid from my teachers, however, was that academic subjects came easily to me and assignments were so simple that I spent much of my time in the classroom daydreaming about the books I was reading and the stories I concocted in my head. I also hid this from my family. I was "the big-headed prawn"—a Chinese term for an absent-minded person—and "the tortoise," a nickname I earned from my difficulty learning new things, tuning in when spoken to, and remembering directions. By middle school, I found it challenging to remember where each classroom was—now there were seven of them!—much less each assignment and exam dates. I began having nightmares about missed deadlines and forgotten tests. My identity began to unravel as I received zeros on pop quizzes and was overwhelmed with the amount of material to learn and tasks to complete. I relied on the good will of teachers to stay on top of deadlines and earn some extra credit. Although my grades reflected a high academic aptitude, I found myself unable to build relationships, cultivate hobbies, and pursue other interests.

By college, I had perfected being the imposter. I projected a calm presence on the surface but felt as though I was frantically treading water. Hidden behind practiced smiles, knowing nods, and a manicured appearance was constant bewilderment. I kept secret the confusion that I felt, every semester, while examining course offerings and learning my new schedule. I kept silent that my undergraduate-level readings were incomprehensible to me—my eyes glazed over the text. I was unable to track any sentence and make sense of the page. Upon graduation, I didn't dare admit that my decision to graduate a year early was to escape the crushing anxiety of having to face yet another year of attempting to survive what seemed to me an endless treacherous ocean. I was tired of pretending: School was just not for me.

The greatest impact was a gaping loneliness that began in childhood and transitioned into many episodes of depression, some with suicidal ideation. Inattentiveness—or the difficulty to "tune in"—meant that I always felt a beat or two behind others. I missed social overtures, could not follow storytelling, did not understand punchlines, and could not remember important details of others' lives the next time I saw them. I always felt awkward around others because while the imposter nodded along pleasantly, my undetected ADHD brain was sorting through an endless barrage of thoughts and stimuli. Feelings of success and pride were nonexistent because I was sure that any accomplishments were actually undeserved—products of luck or others' generosity. Instead, my failures (the failed relationships, the projects I began and left incomplete, the jobs I quietly left after a few months) reinforced my self-view. Gnawing thoughts of ending my life persisted for over a decade.

When I finally sought treatment for ADHD–Inattentive and found the right medication regimen, the transition to my "real" self was immediate. Suddenly, I wasn't a beat behind or a hundred thoughts into the future. I perceived things in real time. I saw and heard things unfold as other typical brains must perceive them: I answered questions, laughed at jokes, and gave my opinions without pause. I transitioned between actions, completed tasks, and met goals without becoming lost in the process. I comprehended readings and put my thoughts on paper on the first attempt. The persistent internal buzz of anxieties and tangents finally quieted.

What could I have accomplished if those around me had recognized my childhood difficulties as a treatable disorder? Were the years of mood and anxiety issues and unmet goals consequences of who I was—or my disorder? These questions linger, but my diagnosis in adulthood has allowed me to reconceptualize the challenges I faced, to experience pride in my accomplishments, and to accept my path as unique to me.

FOUR

What Do You Need to Know about the Causes of ADHD?

When a child has a life-disrupting disorder, it's only natural for parents to ask how and why this problem has befallen the family. ADHD is surely no exception. ADHD is also not protected from the strong inclination to blame parents for whatever ails their children. Despite ever-mounting evidence to the contrary, the myth that "bad parenting" causes ADHD persists, rearing its harmful head in various corners of society (and the media) with alarming regularity. As well, it's quite a jolt, in many cases, for parents to learn that their daughter has real issues in developing self-regulation—which can trigger pessimism and self-blame in both daughter and parents alike.

My main purpose in this chapter, therefore, is to reveal that ADHD has significant roots in your daughter's underlying genetic and biological makeup. In other words, ADHD is not, except in extreme circumstances, the product of "bad parenting." Still, as emphasized in the rest of this book, there's a whole lot that families can do to promote thriving.

In this chapter we'll examine causes of ADHD. My aim is not to provide an in-depth textbook chapter on this complex subject but instead it is to distill what's known about genes in relation to ADHD, along with prenatal and infancy-related processes that can also predict ADHD symptoms. I will also consider the potential for early trauma to either mimic ADHD or compound its symptoms, as such experiences can alter cognitive processing and interpersonal relationships as well as brain functioning.

Please keep in mind, though, that even if parenting is not a direct cause of a child's developing ADHD, family life and parenting styles do matter—a *lot*—if you're raising a girl (or boy) with ADHD. These factors, if not managed optimally, can actually worsen initial ADHD symptoms—or, on the other hand, if handled well, can help your offspring thrive. The same is true for school experiences, as discussed in later chapters. At an even higher level, cultural and societal attitudes toward and acceptance of ADHD can also promote coping and thriving. Chapter 5 elaborates on these themes.

The bottom line is this: It's not biology *or* parenting. It's not biology *or* wider contextual factors. It's always *both,* in combination.

How Biology and Environment Interact

As a helpful overview, consider coronary artery disease, which is a major risk for heart attacks. At a physical level, it involves the buildup of fatty deposits, called *plaques,* inside artery walls. When the arteries that supply blood to one's heart are affected, blood to the heart muscle can be curtailed, potentially triggering heart attacks.

Coronary artery disease runs in families. It does so in part because of genes inherited from parents. Medical scientists are continuing to make discoveries related to patterns of genetic influence that underlie the risk for this truly serious medical condition. Still, genetic vulnerability is not the only causal factor. Across different people, distinct patterns of diet, exercise, lifestyle, exposure to pollution, and additional factors also explain part of the risk for coronary artery disease. Even more, if you are an individual who has strong genetic risk, it truly matters how much you exercise, what kinds of foods you eat, and how you manage stress. In other words, (1) across people, genes explain part of the risk but not the entire risk, and (2) environmental and individual factors and processes can increase or diminish the underlying genetic vulnerability.

ADHD provides a strong parallel here. It runs in families—quite strongly, as discussed below. A whole range of genes, each contributing a small fraction of risk, can add up to make a given individual more likely than other people to show poorly regulated attention and/or high levels of impulsivity and hyperactivity. At the same time, additional causal forces, especially during the prenatal and infancy periods, can trigger ADHD (or add to genetic vulnerability) in other cases. Even more, for individuals with "risky genes," how they learn to regulate impulses and emotions during early childhood—and subsequently adapt to school and manage peer interactions—can either amplify or modify the underlying genetic risk. Once again, effects of genes can be enhanced or modified by processes in the individual's contexts and culture.

Guilt versus Responsibility

In most cases of ADHD, it's the underlying genetics that create the primary risk or vulnerability.

This knowledge might relieve parental guilt: "It's not my parenting—my child was born with a strong risk." Yet for some parents, this news might precipitate a different kind of guilt, as if it's their fault that they have passed on a genetic vulnerability to this neurodevelopmental disorder.

As I emphasize throughout the book, the underlying genes that predispose to ADHD are not fixed, at birth, to lead to a life of impairment and despair. In fact, some of the most "vulnerable" children, related to genes, may also be the most responsive to warm, supportive, encouraging, and rewarding environments.

So, I urge you to do whatever you can to avoid self-blame—that is, to stop beating yourself up, if you've been prone to do so. Simultaneously, however, I emphasize that you still have the core *responsibility* of seeking and obtaining a sound assessment, altering your parenting style, and engaging your daughter in treatment. The fact that you did not cause her ADHD does *not* relieve you of the hard work ahead. To the extent that you can find real strengths in her sometimes different or nontraditional style—and to the extent that you can provide support and rewards, more so than required for most other girls— there is real hope for positive change.

As highlighted throughout this book, several important tasks lie in front of you.

- Pay close attention to how you parent your daughter.
- At the same time, examine patterns of regulation and organization in yourself. In fact, if you're her biological parent, these patterns may well be similar to your daughter's.
- Beyond the best assessment possible, seek the best treatment plan that you can forge with a clinical and educational team. This might include treatment for yourself as her parent.
- Over and above the biological risk that she might "carry," realize that

parenting, schooling, and the general context of the triple bind (see Chapter 3) also matter considerably in relation to your daughter's future functioning.

Drop blame and self-criticism, but don't let yourself off the hook in terms of responsibility and action.

You may not have initially triggered your daughter's ADHD through your parenting style, but you may well be inadvertently perpetuating it—or helping to unleash additional problems by your sometimes futile (and even frantic) attempts to manage both your daughter's stress levels and your own. What it takes, once again, is a kind of radical acceptance of her differences along with a radical commitment to enhancing her strengths and providing support for the areas in which she needs intentional learning.

Is doing all of the above easy? No way. All of us are practically "wired" to take on complete responsibility and blame if our child doesn't fit a narrow definition of what's acceptable. Yet it is now apparent that there is no "normal." All humans differ from one another in a host of ways, emotionally and behaviorally. Those differences can play out quite differently, too, depending on the support or lack thereof one encounters at home, at school or work, and in the general community.

Finally, finding the ways in which your daughter's challenges may actually turn out to be advantages is a major task for all parents, requiring you to accept who she is, encourage her to develop skills and strengths, hold and enforce clear expectations for her behavior, and make necessary changes in your style of parenting and family management.

Let me emphasize one of the points just made: Because ADHD behaviors tend to run in families (often for genetic reasons), it could well be that if your biological daughter has ADHD, one or both parents share some (or even many) of the same traits that she displays. Knowing this might help you forgive yourself and stop at least some of the self-criticism that may be occurring. It might also motivate you to seek

Treatment for your daughter's ADHD is truly a family affair.

assessment and treatment for *yourself*—given that your parenting skills could be compromised by the very kinds of problems in self-regulation you experience, which are parallel to those that your daughter is dealing with.

Genes and ADHD

Genetics is a really complicated topic, and as I said earlier, my goal is not to delve into all that complexity but rather to give you an overview of some of the basics and then tell you what we know about how genes are involved in predisposing a child to ADHD. This understanding is important because it can have a significant impact on how you view your daughter's issues at home, at school, and with peers—and how you go about helping her with them.

As you may remember from high-school biology, each of us is born with 23 pairs of chromosomes, and about half of each pair emanates from our mother's egg cell and the other half from our father's sperm cell. Each chromosome is composed of a lot of DNA. Some "chunks" of DNA are called *genes*. These are the portions that instruct the body to create proteins and other building blocks of our brains and bodies, through messenger RNA and a host of complicated biological processes.

The slight variations between individuals in some genes can lead to differences in traits like hair color, height, skin color, eye color, body type, muscle tone, risk for certain medical diseases (like various cancers or coronary artery disease), cognitive skills, and basic physiological processes. The list continues, with differences in emotion regulation, a host of behavioral and learning tendencies, and mental, neurodevelopmental, and learning conditions.

A huge question in human genetics is which is more important for creating such differences: the genes we're born with or the environments and contexts in which we're raised? Some differences, such as eye color and skin color, are almost entirely the product of genetic differences. But regarding risk for many medical and mental health conditions, as well as behavioral/cognitive/emotional tendencies, it is now well known that environmental influences also can shape where people fall on the spectrum.

How do we even begin to figure this out? The box on pages 95–97 describes the classic methods for doing so. From these methods of the scientific field called *behavioral genetics,* scientists emerge with a percentage, ranging from 0% to 100%, indicating the portion of a given difference between people that comes from their genes as opposed to their environments. This percentage is called *heritability*. One hundred percent means that genes are totally responsible for the differences between people, whereas 0% means that environments and contexts are totally responsible. For most complex traits, the percentage is somewhere in between. The heritability of coronary artery disease, for example, is close to 50%. In other words, a host of studies—family, twin, and adoption, plus investigations of molecular genetics—reveal that about half of the risk for this illness comes from differences in people's genes and about half from differences in environments (including life stress, air quality, the "inner" environment of nutrition, and many more). That is, about half the risk for getting coronary artery disease is genetic.

Does this mean that there's a single gene that contributes to this risk? Not at all. Many genes, each contributing a small part to the "biology" of the size (or flexibility) of one's arteries, or to the body's processes related to "bad cholesterol," or to one's general metabolism, are involved. Obviously, which genes contribute to risk for any condition, including ADHD, is another big question that molecular geneticists, who study actual DNA, are trying to answer.

One thing scientists do know about ADHD is *that its heritability is extremely high, around 80%.* From a host of family, twin, and adoption studies, we know that the reason some people struggle with self-control, sustained attention, and regulating impulses—whereas others are average or high on those traits, showing either decent or excellent self-regulation—is based largely on the different genes they carry.

This perspective is completely different from the way most people think about human behaviors: namely, the view that how individuals act is under the complete control of the parenting they've experienced or their own personal character or "will." For ADHD, there's an added perception that the individual in question should just pay attention, focus, and straighten up: "Just try harder and you'll be fine!" But genes are the main factors that determine how Person A differs from Person B in terms of the behaviors related to ADHD.

Let's consider other mental and neurodevelopmental conditions. The heritability of major depression is about 30% in men and 40% in women. That is, genes matter (slightly more for women than for men) at above-chance levels with respect to the tendency to sink into serious episodes of depression. Yet prenatal factors, parenting, life stress (and how one responds to stress), and a host of other factors matter even more in creating differences in risk for major depression. Schizophrenia's heritability is between 60% and 70%. This often-chronic condition, which entails psychotic behavior (hallucinating, having delusions, losing touch with reality), along with isolation and a retreat from the world, has a substantially high genetic liability. This discovery, too, is a sharp turnaround from several generations ago, when the prevailing view was that parenting styles were the main, if not the only, cause of schizophrenia.

But ADHD's genetic liability is even higher! In fact, the only other major psychiatric conditions with equal or higher heritability scores are bipolar disorder, at over 80%, and autism spectrum disorders, approaching 90%. For all three, genes are the predominant source of the risk. This can matter a lot if you're a parent. In other words, ADHD is one of the most "genetic" conditions a child (or adult) can encounter—a far cry from the common stereotype that it's all about the effects of overly lax or overly harsh parenting, poor schools, or our "device-driven" ways of communicating these days. It means, in fact, that you'll need to be sympathetic to your daughter's differences, not blaming her for her behavioral tendencies, while at the same time working with her and her school in different and important ways.

> *Despite the stereotypes, most of the vulnerability for developing ADHD lies in the genes that an individual inherits.*

Myths about Heritability

From the information just discussed, it might be tempting to conclude that because the heritability of ADHD is around 80%, genes are the only things (or nearly the only things) that matter in producing ADHD in one individual and "neurotypicality" in another. Or to conclude that the only viable ways of treating ADHD are via medications or other biological means, perhaps one day including gene therapy, to replace the aberrant genes. But these conclusions are overstated and even erroneous. I briefly attempt to take on core myths.

Myth 1: Heritability is destiny. We are all born with our full complement of DNA and of the genes located "inside" that DNA. But experiences in our bodies and in the outside world activate when different genes express themselves, at different times and in different parts of the body, including the brain. *Epigenetics* refers to the intricate processes by which contextual factors are crucial for "switching on" certain genes.

Furthermore, even certain conditions that are 100% heritable can be modified by nongenetic means. For example, phenylketonuria (PKU) is a rare disorder, resulting from a single gene inherited in a baby, with one recessive allele of that gene inherited from each parent. In other words, the only way one gets PKU is from these alleles of this single gene. When PKU occurs, the baby and developing individual cannot metabolize the amino acid phenylalanine—leading to brain dysfunction and intellectual disability. However, if this condition is recognized at birth and the child is placed on a phenylalanine-free diet, the later IQ is often 100, completely average. In this case, the nutritional environment inside the child's body can outweigh the single genetic problem that triggers the disease.

Myth 2. High heritability means that defective or "bad" genes are at play in psychiatric and neurodevelopmental conditions. In some cases (as with PKU, just discussed), a single gene is harmful to human health and functioning. But for most medical and psychiatric conditions, there are hundreds or even thousands of genes interacting in complex combinations that produce heritable risk. And many of those genes may have helped to shape behaviors, in human history, that were adaptive then but are less so now. Regarding ADHD, genes predicting impulsive/"explorer" behaviors in the past may have pushed some humans to migrate to new lands—but in our postindustrial world of classrooms and long periods of enforced sitting, those genes may predispose people to a diagnosis of ADHD.

Myth 3: Strong heritability means that traits can't be altered. Actually, traits can change in a population! How tall you are, relative to others, is extremely heritable—90% or higher. Thousands of genes interact together to provide the "ceiling" of your ultimate adult stature, and these genes matter far more than environments in determining where you fall on the height chart. Even so, all of us are several inches taller than our great-grandparents or great-great grandparents, on average. Why? Not because of massive gene mutations—the effects of those would take many generations to appear. Instead, largely because of our diets (more protein, certain hormones, and the like), the heights of the whole population have increased.

Let's consider ADHD in this light: It could well be the case that rates are rising, particularly in high-achievement, postmodern cultures that press for ever-earlier academic skills, or the advent of iPhones and social media (requiring very short bursts of attention), or our increasingly fast-paced world. But even so, the reasons some people develop ADHD but most do not, today, are still related much more to genes than to contexts. So, I highlight two implications: (1) There's the hope that we can create environments that help everyone self-regulate better, and (2) it's time to drop self-blame for the causes of your daughter's ADHD.

Myth 4: Heritability applies to everyone in the population to the same extent. Scores on intelligence tests (IQ tests) are moderately heritable, across the population. Genes have a real contribution to differences in such scores across people. But the heritability of IQ scores is not uniform. That is, for those in the highest income bracket, IQ has a heritability that is huge, approaching 90%. But for those in the lowest income bracket, heritability of IQ is not much above 10%.

How can this be? The answer can get technical, but the principle is quite important. Basically, if kids grow up with all sorts of socioeconomic advantages, including good diets, stimulating home environments, and high-quality schools, the only major factor predicting better versus worse IQ scores pertains to heritable (genetic) differences in their ability to process information quickly, their conceptual abilities, and the like. This is because contextual factors don't really vary all that much for the wealthiest, meaning that genetic factors are the key determinants of differences in IQ. Yet if kids grow up in poverty, many influential contextual factors play a role: pollution in the air, less-than-adequate nutrition, low cognitive stimulation at home, crowded and poorly funded schools, trauma from neighborhood violence, and the like. These environmental factors far outweigh any effects of genes on differences in IQ scores.

The bottom line: Just because a condition, like ADHD, shows high heritability does *not* mean that families, schools, communities, and individuals are unimportant. Far from it!

Genes Linked to ADHD—and Delayed Brain Maturation

The multiple genes that predict risk for ADHD, acting together in ways that science has only just begun to understand, code for a huge number of brain structures, brain growth, and brain connections. It will take much more research to pinpoint the highly complex "mapping" of genes onto brain development—and how divergent life experiences may also shape development—regarding ADHD. The same is true for a host of other mental and neurodevelopmental disorders. The box on pages 97–98 provides a few remarkable facts about the brain and its development.

An incredible set of research findings has proven highly relevant for ADHD. Some 20 years ago, a major study took place, using 223 children with ADHD (including 141 boys and 82 girls) and exactly the same number of typically developing children (with the same ratio of 141 boys to 82 girls). This longitudinal study used sophisticated brain-scanning technology, which mapped the size (thickness) of the brain's cortex over the course of development. As explained in the box, the cortex is the outermost layer of the brain, which contains brain cells (neurons), each of which sends huge numbers of projections to other brain regions. The key focus has been the prefrontal area of the brain, just behind your forehead, which is essential for self-control, planning, and regulation of impulses.

In the typically developing children, the prefrontal cortex reached its maximum thickness at around age 7. But in the boys and girls with ADHD, the maximum thickness did not appear until three or more years later—after age 10. This landmark finding therefore signaled a crucial lag in brain development in a large sample of children with ADHD.

Just think of it: Largely because of genetic differences between youth with ADHD and those without, brain development—in the crucial region and networks linked with self-control—is delayed (or "immature") for those with ADHD, by a considerable gap. In follow-up studies of the same sample, the gap continued into late adolescence, a period when the cortex continues to mature by pruning, actually becoming thinner as it gets more efficient. This thinning process, too, was delayed in the ADHD sample by several years.

> *In both girls and boys with ADHD, brain development is delayed by about three years compared to children without ADHD.*

Most of the sample in this study had the combined form of ADHD, including both inattention and hyperactivity-impulsivity. And boys did outnumber girls (although the number of girls was relatively large). Still, the results are truly provocative. In fact, recall from Chapter 1 that one of the many names for ADHD throughout the 20th century was the *immaturity syndrome,* because of the observation that children with ADHD often acted several years younger than their chronological age. Now MRI scans reveal that such immaturity may well occur with respect to brain development.

So, here's what I ask you to do now. Take a long look at your daughter, the one whose inattentive behavior patterns may have prompted her teachers, and you, to assume that she simply doesn't care about her schoolwork or is somehow hopelessly unmotivated. Or the one whose stubborn, defiant, and impulsive actions lead you to believe that she must be asserting her will to undermine your authority. All this can be exasperating, to say the least. You may ask: Why can't she be more like other girls? Why has my relationship with her deteriorated to this point? What did I do wrong?

But for reasons beyond the socialization and parenting she's received, she may well have a brain that is several years behind the development of other kids' brains—especially in the frontal lobes and their massive connections with other brain regions, which are central to the display of self-regulation. Of course, it may be a shock to learn of this possibility, which might even make you feel helpless as a parent. Yet be assured that the material throughout the rest of this book—on obtaining treatment and working hard on setting up home and home–school programs, as well as the potential for medication treatments—can give you skills in helping your daughter's thriving and eventual independence.

> Knowing that your daughter's ADHD symptoms flow largely from her genes can transform your attitude toward why she behaves the way she does.

Genes and Environments

Even though ADHD is around 80% heritable, this doesn't mean that environments have no impact on how well your daughter functions in daily life, now or in the future. Here's why.

The methods used to understand heritability—family, twin, and adoption studies—operate under the assumption that the effects of genes and environments are completely separate and independent. In other words, it's either genes or environments. But in biological families, this assumption just isn't accurate. A child born to and raised by biological parents (1) shares half of her genes with her mother and half with her father, while (2) she lives with them and is parented by them. But the parents' own ways of raising her are in part shaped by the very genes they carry, which they have also transmitted to her. In the case of ADHD, the daughter's inattention and impulsivity levels are therefore shaped by genes *and* by her parents' ways of socializing her, *at the same time.*

Even more, this girl may well act in such a way (shaped largely by her genes) as to elicit her parents' frustration, which is already higher than typical because of their genes. As you can see, a vicious cycle is now unfolding. Again, where the influence of genes and environment is concerned, it's *both–and,* not either–or.

At a more technical level, I mentioned earlier the concept of *epigenetics,* which signifies that certain genes come to life (or,

> *Whether genes or environment cause ADHD is not either–or but both–and.*

more technically, are "expressed") only when a change in the body's physiology or a change in the surrounding environment activates them. Once again, genes and environments work in concert.

Even more, when difficult life experiences piggyback on top of genetic/biological risk, particularly troublesome outcomes are highly likely to occur. On the other hand, certain truly supportive and protective environments may lead to especially favorable outcomes when acting on certain kinds of genes. In other words, these genes or gene combinations may not be inherently risky—rather, they may be highly susceptible to the influence of either maladaptive or extremely positive environments (see the box on pages 90–91 for illustration through the metaphor of orchids and dandelions).

The bottom line: Just because your daughter's extremes of disorganization, poor self-regulation, or impulse-control problems are likely to be, in large part, linked to the genes she's inherited does *not* mean that parenting and schooling are unimportant or irrelevant. In fact, they may well be even *more* important than is the case for a youngster lacking such genetic risk. I provide more on this fascinating and crucial topic in Chapter 5.

Prenatal and Early-Life Risk Factors

Other biological processes during early development can also lead to later ADHD. The developing brain is nothing short of miraculous. Little wonder that exposure of such a "brain-in-progress" to poisons or toxins before birth, or during the first years of life, could prove to be highly consequential to the development of issues in self-regulation, attention and organization, impulse control, and more. I present the brief information below because it may help you contextualize and better understand early factors potentially related to your daughter's ADHD and, once again, help alleviate some of the self-blame you may be carrying around regarding how you interact with her.

Orchids versus Dandelions

When the fields of behavioral genetics, and then molecular genetics, gained traction in the 20th century, much of the thinking centered on the kinds of mutations, or "bad genes," that could lead to problems in learning, behavior, and performance. In fact, early behavioral genetics studies were often incredibly reductionistic, asserting without evidence that deviant genes were the root of many social ills. The findings were inherently racist and sexist; they were used in both the United States and Nazi Germany to legitimize sterilization in women and horrible abuses of rights, including extermination, of many religious, sexual, and racial minorities (as well as of individuals with intellectual disabilities and mental disorders).

Even in more modern and far more rigorous science, there is still a tendency to relate any negative outcome to a deviant, bad, or pathological gene or set of genes. But there is an alternative interpretation that could be radically useful to parents and others trying to help girls (and boys) with ADHD thrive.

In what is technically called the *differential susceptibility* model, the core idea is that genes or gene combinations that make individuals vulnerable to problematic traits or disorders do *not* inevitably lead to negative outcomes. The newer vision is that certain genotypes are instead highly sensitive to the input from contexts and environments, whether for good or for ill.

An excellent metaphor for this theory comes from the recent, important book by my colleague W. Thomas Boyce of the University of California, San Francisco. In fact, the book's very title, *The Orchid and the Dandelion*, spells out this contention. Dandelions are hearty weeds: They grow anywhere and seemingly everywhere, seemingly impervious to climate, soil composition, altitude, and the like. Orchids, on the other hand, require delicate and assiduous care. If they don't receive it, they do not thrive, but when they do, their flowers are magnificent.

Summing up his own research and that of many other scientists, Boyce conveys that the underlying genes believed to signal vulnerability to difficult outcomes are actually acutely sensitive to context. *This means that certain environments and contexts can be geared toward helping the "vulnerable" child thrive.* Under enriched circumstances, in fact, this child may well turn out better than most of the dandelions making up the majority of their peers—and certainly better than children with the same genotype who do not benefit from the enriching circumstances.

It's too early to tell whether this is true for ADHD. Yet our lab has found at least some evidence in favor of this view (see Chapter 5). The take-home message is that conditions like ADHD do not inevitably lead to negative outcomes—and that environments may actually be particularly important for what are often considered to be high-risk genes.

Alcohol

As the result of research conducted over a number of decades, it's now clear that when a pregnant mother ingests alcohol, later effects on development are highly noteworthy. If a mother drinks repeatedly, and particularly when binge drinking is involved, the baby may be born with full *fetal alcohol syndrome*. But even moderate or occasional drinking can lead to *fetal alcohol spectrum disorders,* which involve the very kinds of attentional, impulse-control-related, and hyperactive behaviors that are part of the ADHD spectrum. Real problems in learning, social interactions, and family functioning can result. In cases of adoption, it could be that one reason some biological mothers needed to give up their child for adoption had to do with prenatal drinking or substance abuse. There's nothing to be done to "undo" such a history—but there's plenty to do to help your daughter thrive.

Interestingly, the pregnant women (or girls) most likely to engage in drinking could be those with impulse-control problems or the kinds of attention problems leading them to have become disengaged with school. In other words, it could well be the case that the genes that predict ADHD in a mother—the same genes she passes on to her offspring—also predict drinking during pregnancy, which can further induce ADHD-related symptoms. This is another example of how genes and contextual factors (in this case, prenatal alcohol) can sum together.

Smoking

Prenatal smoking of cigarettes, or vaping, or other forms of ingesting nicotine (and the many toxic chemicals associated with nicotine use via cigarettes) are also associated with both ADHD symptoms and oppositional/defiant symptoms in the developing child. Here, however, it is still unclear whether it's the explicit exposure to the nicotine and the other chemicals involved—versus the genes in the mother that may predict her propensity to smoke or vape—that is the main culprit.

There's no room to review the fairly limited knowledge of the effects of other, often illicit drugs ingested by pregnant women with respect to ADHD-related outcomes. Should you choose to have more children, however, it makes sense to refrain from smoking and other drugs while pregnant.

Toxic Chemicals

Some chemicals, like lead, are another risk factor. In particular, lead that an infant or toddler may "mouth" from crumbling paint chips, may drink if water enters the building from lead pipes, or may breathe in from the air from old-style gasoline fumes can result in later problems such as poor concentration and learning, impulsive behavior, and overactivity. Even though this hypothesis was doubted in the middle of the last century—and even though industries promoting lead fought the growing findings for years—there is little doubt that the effects can be real. Importantly, it's not just extremely high levels of lead in one's bloodstream, called *lead poisoning,* that can trigger ADHD symptoms, but far lower levels that are typically not deemed as poisonous. Such findings are part of the reason that ADHD is no longer considered a middle-class, male issue these days—as environmental lead is particularly prevalent in lower-class neighborhoods and appears to affect the developing brains of boys and girls similarly.

If you're the parent of an infant or young child, whether their suspected of having ADHD or not, it's a great idea to check paint in your house, the kinds of pipes bringing in water, and the levels of lead and other contaminants in the air near your home.

Less information is available about additional chemicals, like pesticides—or phthalates (that is, chemicals in plastics and their derivatives, found in home products and many cosmetics)—but research suggests that they could well be linked to the development of ADHD symptoms, or in some cases autism spectrum disorders. In another example of how genes and environmental influences can act in combination, researchers speculate that children with genetic vulnerability to ADHD may be particularly susceptible to the neurodevelopmental effects of such chemicals.

Prescription (or Over-the-Counter) Medications

There are a great many daily medicines that people, including pregnant people, take for a range of health-related issues, along with prescribed medical and psychiatric medications that they may need. To sum up the potential effects on developing children (which could fill at least a chapter), some medications during pregnancy are not safe at all (for example, lithium for bipolar disorder, which has known negative effects on the developing fetus). For many others, there is *some* evidence of potential risk, but not enough evidence to suggest that the pregnant person should absolutely stop the medication they are taking. For example, serious depression during pregnancy, if untreated, may well have major downstream effects on the developing child. There are too many cases where insufficient data exist to make a clear decision. The bottom line here is that if you're pregnant and wondering about which medications to continue or discontinue for the duration of the pregnancy, *ask your doctor.*

Low Birth Weight

Research has shown that being born below 5½ pounds (defined as *low birth weight*)—or, at more extreme levels, *very low birth weight* or *extremely low birth weight* (under about 3½ or 2½ pounds, respectively)—can predict a host of physical, neurodevelopmental, and behavioral problems for the developing child. Included here are many of the symptoms of ADHD. The reasons are many: A crucial one is that preterm and/or low-birth-weight babies may experience breakage of blood vessels toward the front of the brain, leading to later learning disorders, Tourette syndrome, cerebral palsy, or ADHD.

Note that, over the past decades, many babies born at well-below-average birth weights, who would almost never have survived in earlier eras, are placed in neonatal intensive care units, which can keep them alive. In fact, one contributor (though probably a small one, overall) to the increased rates of ADHD in our current world is that more and more babies born at low birth weights now survive because of far superior neonatal care facilities.

> *Even the most severe risk factors may be overcome by recognition, accurate assessment, and treatment.*

Does all this mean, though, that babies born at below-average weights inevitably develop ADHD or other disorders? The answer is no. My own research team knows of girls born at incredibly low birth weights, several decades ago, who have (1) received intensive treatment during childhood and (2) gone on to college and graduate education, with wonderful lives. The lesson is clear: No single risk factor inevitably dooms a young person with ADHD to a life of serious impairment.

Trauma and Abuse

A child who experiences severe deprivation during the early years has a well-above-average chance of developing (1) a lack of meaningful attachment bonds to caregivers, which can presage later relationship problems and (2) both inattention and overactivity. A clear example is found in follow-up studies of children placed in horrifically understaffed, custodial orphanages in Eastern Europe during the latter part of the 20th century. These important findings reveal that severe early deprivation can result in patterns of behavior similar to those in children with more typical cases of ADHD.

Also, in the United States and many other countries, early child neglect and child abuse can predispose children to the experience of the world as an unpredictable place, to lapses in attention, and to patterns of impulsive behavior. In general, acts of physical abuse predict aggression in the child, whereas sexual abuse can lead to a damaged sense of self, low motivation, and anxiety/depression. In children experiencing such forms of trauma, especially those who get placed in foster care during early years, separating what's "ADHD" from aftereffects of trauma is an extremely difficult task, as noted in Chapter 2, where I covered thorough diagnostic assessments.

> It's clear that ADHD is not one single entity. Multiple roads can lead to Rome.

Often, it's not a matter of "definite ADHD" versus "definite trauma." Adverse and traumatic childhood experiences may well emanate from parents who themselves experience serious symptoms of ADHD, often compounded by a lack of financial resources, substance abuse, and/or their own childhood trauma. Even more, research from my own laboratory shows that girls with ADHD who have additionally experienced physical abuse, sexual abuse, or neglect display a far higher risk for self-harm than girls with ADHD who have not had such histories (see also Chapter 3). Quite often, once again, it's *both–and* rather than *either–or*.

What is the take-home message for you? If you are an adoptive or foster parent, you may be able to learn some, or even a considerable amount, about the status of your daughter's biological parent, including the potential for early traumatic experiences. If such evidence exists, it may be advisable to gain understanding of "trauma-informed" care (see Resources at the end of this book). It's also particularly helpful to emphasize positive contingencies and consequences in work with such children.

● ● ●

In Chapter 5, I take up the topic of parenting in explicit detail. I hope this chapter's main message has been clear: The research data we have on what causes ADHD and what is likely to contribute to your daughter's outcome indicate that you should reduce your self-blame but at the same time dedicate yourself to understanding your daughter better and pursuing positive change. Chapter 5 develops this theme further, with information about parenting practices, styles, and philosophies that can help your daughter thrive.

Research Methods Used to Understand the Influence of Genes on Differences among People

Research in behavioral genetics uses patterns of family relationships to estimate the relative roles of genes and environments in explaining why people differ in cognitive performance, behavioral traits, medical conditions, or psychiatric diagnoses. The methods typically require large numbers of participants. Here are the three primary types of research methods.

Family Studies

Based on animal research and then applied to humans, *family studies* (sometimes called *pedigree studies*) assume that biological relatives are more likely to "share" a trait or disorder than nonrelatives—and the more closely related they are, the more the trait or disorder will be shared. In a classic example, schizophrenia has a prevalence of about 1% in the population, so a nonrelative of a person with schizophrenia has about a 1% chance of developing the disorder. But biological relatives have a greater chance: Having a brother or sister with schizophrenia means the risk raises to about 10%, having one biological parent with schizophrenia raises it to 12%, and having both biological parents elevates the risk to between 35% and 40%.

Twin Studies

Twin studies are basically an extension of family studies. Fraternal twins are siblings—sharing, on average, half their genes with each other—who happen to be born at the same time, as two fertilized eggs develop simultaneously in the mother's womb. If one fraternal twin has schizophrenia, the chances that the other will develop it are about 15%, slightly higher than the rate for nontwin siblings. But identical twins are essentially clones, sharing virtually 100% of genes, as they emanate from the same fertilized egg that splits at conception. If one identical twin has schizophrenia, the chances for the other are around 50%. Thus, genes again appear to play a large role.

In fact, if you like a bit of math, one basic way to estimate heritability is to take the chances that identical twins are *concordant* (sharing the same trait or condition), then subtract the parallel rate for fraternal twins, and multiply that difference by 2. For schizophrenia, one would take 50% minus 15%—that is, 35%—then multiply by 2 to get 70%, which is remarkably close to the heritability for this disorder calculated in more sophisticated ways.

The rates for ADHD are different values, because ADHD is more prevalent overall than schizophrenia. Yet the underlying patterns are highly similar, yielding a heritability between 75% and 85%. In short, the more genes you share with a relative, the stronger the chances that you'll both have ADHD-related traits as well as diagnosable ADHD.

But there's a huge catch to family and twin studies. Close relatives share not only genes but also their environments. And identical twins are likely to be treated more similarly than fraternal twins. So, although family studies and twin studies suggest strong genetic roots for schizophrenia, ADHD, autism, and bipolar disorder, along with more moderate heritability estimates for other conditions, it could be the case that it's their similar environments that are the culprit, not just similar genes.

One solution (though an extremely rare one in practice) would be to find identical twins separated at birth, then subsequently raised in different adoptive homes, even in different geographic locations. The few studies of this type have shown some real similarities between such twins in terms of certain personality traits—but there are simply not large-enough samples to be of relevance to most mental or neurodevelopmental disorders.

Adoption Studies

A third way of trying to separate genes and environments is through *adoption studies*. Here, researchers look for greater "sharedness" of traits or disorders in one's adoptive relatives (including those in the same family involved in child rearing) versus biological relatives (who share genes but no personal interactions). This method is not perfect: There is no random selection of families who are eligible for adopting children. Still, adoption studies have a greater chance of separating genetic and environmental effects. Overall, they echo the findings of family and twin studies with respect to supporting substantial heritability for ADHD.

Finally, remember that in the real world, genes and environments are interconnected. Because of the linkages between genes and contexts, some of the more advanced mathematics in calculating heritability may actually overstate, at least to some extent, the role of genes.

A Brief Overview of How the Brain Develops— and What Happens with ADHD

The area of study called *developmental neuroscience* is growing quickly. A few headline concepts and facts may prove helpful in understanding what occurs during typical brain development—and why it's important that this process is delayed, on average, in ADHD.

First, the brain is the most complex entity in the known universe. Weighing in at not much over 3 pounds, it comprises, in adults, approximately 100 billion brain cells (called *neurons*), most of which interconnect with large numbers of other neurons (sometimes thousands of others). Neurons send electric impulses down their long projections, called *axons;* a chemical (called *a neurotransmitter*) is then released, which causes a subsequent electrical current to flow down the next neuron in the chain. What an intricate dance! If one considers the numbers of interconnections across neurons in our brains, the number is on the order of 100 *trillion*. To say that this is "complex" is one of the understatements of the century.

Second, during the prenatal period—the time between the formation of the neural tube, the precursor to the brain, and then the brain itself, up to the baby's birth, an eight-month span—many thousands of neurons develop, *every second*. That is, 8,000 or so, *every second, continuously, for 35 weeks!* This fact is nothing short of miraculous. Even more, connections between and among neurons begin to form as well, and these number many more thousands each second.

Third, babies are in fact born with about double the 100 billion neurons that exist in adult brains. During the brain's continuing development over the first several years of life, many billions of neurons that do not develop viable connections with other neurons essentially die off. This process is called *pruning,* assuring that only those well-connected neurons in the brain stay functional.

Fourth, the outermost layer of the brain is the *cortex* (the origin of this word refers to "bark"—that is, the thin, outermost part of a tree trunk). Another name for the cortex is *gray matter,* because the cell body (including the nucleus) of a neuron is gray colored—and millions of cell bodies are packed throughout each tiny segment of the cortex. The long projections from each cell body—*axons*—travel through the brain to connect with other cell bodies. These constitute the white matter, as axons are coated with white-colored myelin, which helps to speed up the electric current running through them.

In typical development, after initial pruning during the first couple of years of life, the neurons in the cortex proliferate, thickening it before a peak of thickness is reached at around 7 years old. This is especially true in the prefrontal cortex, as described in the main text, where executive functions and self-regulation are undergirded by the fantastic number of connections with other brain regions. Then, throughout later childhood, adolescence, and the early years of adulthood, the cortex reprunes—again, becoming more efficient—until reaching its "final" levels in the mid-20s.

Yet in the landmark study by Philip Shaw and colleagues, at the National Institutes of Health, it was discovered that, on average, boys and girls with ADHD do not attain their maximum prefrontal cortical thickness until age 10 or after. Moreover, the next stage of repruning in adolescence is also several years late for many people with ADHD. No one is quite sure whether these delays emanate from genetic "programming" directly, from the role of certain experiences in slowing brain maturation, or from some combination. But the core point is that the apparent behavioral and emotional immaturity of many individuals with ADHD appears to have a neural basis. The same pattern is found in additional research that examines not only the thickness of the prefrontal cortex but also the development of interconnected brain circuits across wide regions of the brain.

On the basis of such fascinating research, it is clearly not tenable for anyone to claim that girls and boys with ADHD are simply lazy, or not trying hard enough. Or for anyone (including yourself) to blame you: "Bad parenting" is *not* responsible for ADHD. You now have a lot of information you can use to educate others to this important fact to whatever extent you wish to do so. And taking blame out of the picture can free your energy for the hard work of pursuing important changes in your daughter's home and school life.

FIVE

Principles for Parenting a Girl with ADHD

In Chapter 4 I made a point that might appear to contradict what we know about the causes of ADHD in girls (and boys): Parenting matters. Please let me clarify. No, how you parent your daughter doesn't *cause* the disorder. But parenting *does* contribute greatly to outcomes for girls with ADHD. Despite the biological realities underlying ADHD, parenting practices are essential to changing the trajectory for your daughter and her condition.

How parenting contributes to a happy, healthy future for your child and exactly what to keep in mind to promote your daughter's welfare is the focus of this and the following chapters. In this chapter I present current science related to the essential concept of parenting. I'll explain the fundamentals of parent–child attachment and analyze the main dimensions of parenting behaviors—responsiveness/warmth and control/demandingness. I'll also get into other key parenting practices of real relevance as your daughter gets older: monitoring, consistency (within a given parent and between parents), and "fit" (that is, the realignment of parenting philosophies to different children). All of this forms a foundation for the following chapters, where I lay out in more detail the kinds of practical, evidence-based strategies that can help your daughter with ADHD thrive at home, at school, and in the world at large. In fact, without some core background regarding the key components of parenting, many of these practical strategies may appear to come out of the blue.

Attachment

Let's begin at the beginning. When a baby is born, and even before (during the prenatal period), most parents have real hopes and expectations of forming a close relationship with her, full of responsiveness and care. On the other hand, for a host of difficult reasons—general life stress, family crowding, problematic issues in early relationships with their own parents, or competing economic or psychological needs—some parents may not be as available and responsive as the baby or young child requires.

Overall, the quality of the bond between a newborn and her parent is termed *attachment*. Furthermore, it's not just in the first months or even years of life that the attachment bond is important. Close attachments are essential across the life span.

Babies are completely dependent on their caregivers for survival. Don't think, though, that young children are simply passive recipients of inputs from their environments. Instead, babies differ from one another in their basic, biologically driven ways of showing emotions and behaving in the world (sometimes called *temperament*). And they are active observers and synthesizers of what they perceive in terms of safety and security, well before they can talk. Indeed, babies have a kind of "sixth sense" about how responsive their parents are during the crucial early months of development.

Let's take a broader view. Secure attachment bonds are essential for any primate species, particularly humans. After all, primates are typically not as large, strong, or fast as potential predators. And primate babies need long periods of development during which they must (1) be kept safe and (2) learn the essential skills necessary to survive and thrive. Human babies, in particular, need to learn, from families and cultures, the many cognitive and socioemotional strategies needed to thrive and contribute to their community.

During the early days and months of life, babies put out distress calls when their needs are overwhelming. It's hard to think of a stronger tug on your heartstrings—or patience—than the piercing sound of an infant's cries when hungry or tired. Simultaneously, parents are particularly attuned to respond to those signals. Thank goodness (and natural selection) that nearly all adults see babies as adorable. In other words, especially if the baby is ours, we feel closely bonded to them, especially when social smiles emerge at a few months of age. Without all this, no humans would be around today. The youngest members of our species require huge amounts of attention and regular, sensitive caregiving. Not "perfect" amounts—no parent can be superhuman—but regular and adequate.

Although most parents provide ample comfort and nurture to their infants and toddlers, yielding a secure parent–child attachment, others may not be as able to do so. Babies sense such ambivalence and distance. Over time, young children with insecure attachments are less likely to actively explore their growing worlds—and may be at risk for problems in social relationships as they grow older, as well as for depression and even aggressive behavior.

At the extremes of a parent's distance or negativity, there could be trauma—either neglect of core needs or instances of abuse. As discussed in Chapter 4, in some cases trauma and abuse can lead to patterns of behavior resembling ADHD. On the other hand, an insecure attachment between parent and baby is not, in and of itself, a core causal factor for ADHD.

If this is the case, why bring up the topic of attachment at all? The reason is that the strength of a bond between you and your child has a *lot* to do with how well your family will be able to promote the strengths of your daughter and engage in treatment with her. Indeed, interventions for ADHD (especially in childhood) rarely consist of one-on-one therapy between the youth and a counselor or therapist. Rather, the whole family needs to be engaged in ways of changing communication and interaction patterns, getting teachers and school officials involved, and supporting medication treatment if it's prescribed. If the parent–child relationship doesn't have at least some trust and good will, there's a strong chance that progress will be minimal.

For example, parent management training is one of the core evidence-based treatments for ADHD. But how can you, as a parent, deliver "positives" to your daughter (or, on the other hand, sustain negative consequences) unless you and she have an underlying connection? Before many parent management programs begin to establish reward charts or teach parents to use negative consequences like time-out for their offspring with ADHD, initial weeks are devoted to reestablishing a positive bond between parent and child. In short, limits and negative consequences won't have a good chance of helping unless a positive connection between you and your daughter is established—or is in the process of being reestablished.

An important point to remember at all times is that, despite the nearly inevitable stresses and strains related to family interactions when ADHD is involved, searching for and relishing your daughter's competencies, working on strengths rather than dwelling on weaknesses, and forming a stronger family bond are crucial parts of effective treatment.

Think of it this way: Your daughter with ADHD may well have been, in her initial months of life, more intense, or less attentive to you or others, than other babies (including her siblings if she has any). It may have been more difficult for you, as her parent, to experience the same consistent bond that you did with your other children, because she was just, well, more difficult. And as emphasized in Chapter 4, her brain development across childhood and adolescence may well be slower than that of other children. It may be harder to maintain a close bond with a child who doesn't display the easygoing temperament or timetable of maturation that many other babies, toddlers, and children display.

But it's never too late to work on regaining a sense of attachment security with your daughter (or son) with ADHD. Research shows that even in the presence of insecure attachment bonds early in life, once parents can "get their acts together" to become more stable sources of support, receive therapy themselves, or regain stability at home, more secure bonds can emerge. These predict better life outcomes. In fact, working toward a responsive bond is still crucial even when your daughter is a teenager and beyond. Given the long period of human development into maturity, it's worth the hard work involved to forgive, understand, reframe, and seek out and cherish the moments of closeness that can truly help with efforts toward change, despite periods of frustration that can be part of the picture.

> Strong attachment bonds form the foundation for the whole family's support of a girl with ADHD.

As highlighted below, kids and teens with ADHD have a real penchant for annoying (or at least testing the patience of) teachers and peers (as well as their parents!). This is all the more reason why you, as your daughter's parent, should work to understand her better, to accept some of her differences, and above all, to support her as she (often erratically) navigates through her classroom, with her peers, and in her wider settings to find her standing. There's really no substitute for a caring, accepting, yet still pushing-for-positive-change parenting bond to help her weather the storms that so many girls (and boys) with ADHD encounter.

Parenting Styles

As children mature, there are countless tasks that parents must perform, countless emotional reactions and responses that parents display (and model for their children), countless interactions with teachers/schools and in the neighborhood, and countless situations that require limits and/or discipline.

For many decades scientists have tried to organize the multitude of parenting attitudes, emotional responses, and practices found in families around the world into fundamental types or dimensions. Across many cultures, two core aspects have emerged from compiling and analyzing hundreds of relevant studies.

Two Fundamental Dimensions

The box on pages 104–105 gives a brief overview of the ways in which researchers and clinicians attempt to measure parenting behaviors and styles.

Responsiveness/Warmth

First, parents fall on a spectrum related to their sense of connection, including responsiveness and warmth, with their child. Also involved here is their fundamental acceptance of the child. On the extreme low end of this dimension, parents may even wish that the child had not been born: They show little if any warmth and may even be hostile toward being that child's parent. On the high end, parents seem to burst at the seams with joy over having this child—and work toward accepting the child's growth as well as appreciating and loving the act of being her parent. Imagine that this dimension, typically called *responsiveness/warmth*, is a horizontal axis, on which the underlying feelings, attitudes, and behaviors grow steadily stronger, moving from left to right. The figure on page 105 shows this dimension as the horizontal *x*-axis.

You might pause for a moment and appraise where you believe you fall on this dimension. Regarding your daughter, were you and are you still joyful over having her in your life? Do you still relish her new discoveries, with your sense of good will toward her sufficient to overcome the inevitable challenges of parenting? Do you let her know, through praise, hugs, and expectations for success, how you feel? Or were things difficult enough, back when she was born, that you perceived her as a source of strife or problems? Alternatively, has your initial enthusiasm given way to frequent frustration, regret, and pessimism, above and beyond day-to-day ups and downs? Does it feel as if the majority of interactions between you two are argumentative, hostile, or sarcastic?

Sometimes it's helpful simply to list the ways in which you show (or would like to show) warmth to your daughter. A plethora of physical affection might, over time, give way to high-fives, or points on a reward chart, or more subtle indicators of the pleasure you find in parenting her. Many overt and more

How Do We Measure Parenting Practices and Styles?

Clinicians and scientists have long wondered how to assess parenting in optimal and valid ways. Here's a quick review.

First, many self-report scales and checklists exist for parents. On these, a parent appraises how much or how often she or he engages in various parenting practices and conveys fundamental attitudes about parenting. These scales are convenient and, by definition, don't require observations of parenting in a clinic or the real world. On the other hand, there's a major issue. Except for some parenting scales on which it's not entirely clear that the item signifies "good" versus "bad" parenting, there's a tendency for many parents to overrate their skills and strengths. How many parents, in fact, will admit that they are inconsistent, overly punitive, or cold with their child? Some clearly do, but additional sources of information are often extremely helpful.

Second, for children who can read and write, there are parallel scales, related to the same core parenting practices as found on parent-reported scales. Intriguingly, for preschoolers, creative measures have been devised, such as having them watch a puppet show within which the characters act out several types of parenting—and having the child speak about whether her own home interactions are similar. Children's reports of parenting grow in sophistication as youth emerge into their teens, but even earlier, they can provide an important counterpoint to parents' reports about themselves.

Third, after observing family interactions in a therapy room, clinicians can put together narrative reports or complete scales dealing with the kinds of parenting they have observed. An advantage here is that trained and experienced clinicians should have wisdom and objectivity. Yet some wonder how representative the family's interactions in a therapist's office truly are of their behavior patterns and interchanges at home.

Finally, clinicians and researchers can videotape clinic/lab observations, so that trained observers can later code the interactions for microbehaviors as well as more global appraisals. Although typically impractical, some of the best information on parenting has emerged from in-home observations or in-home audio recordings of interaction patterns. The latter can be expensive and intrusive, but much of the information presented in this chapter is based on such work.

As is the case for many other aspects of measurement in psychology and mental health, there is far from perfect agreement across these sources.

Ideally, putting together different measurement tools can help to yield a clearer picture.

Note: It is vitally important to consider the role of *culture* in all of the preceding measures—and in interpreting parenting behaviors and practices in general. Does the standard for upper-middle-class majority families, typically thought of as authoritative parenting, pertain to Asian American families, who may value deference to parental authority, more restricted emotional displays, and a strong push toward academic success? Or to Black families, who may for historical reasons favor a more authoritarian style? Or to Latinx families, often comprising larger rather than small nuclear families? And beyond culture per se, some believe that the degree of acculturation in family members is of clear importance.

No one said that parenting is an easy topic. In fact, assuming that one size or one style of parenting fits all children across all cultures equally well is almost certainly misguided.

Chart of the Two Key Parenting Dimensions, with Four Parenting Styles

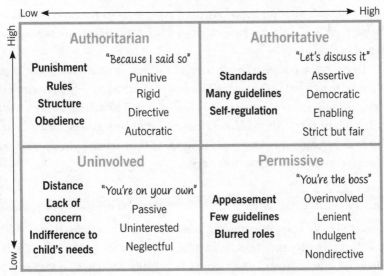

subtle means of showing your daughter how much you value and even treasure her exist.

Control/Demandingness

The second core dimension pertains to the amounts of control, demandingness, authority, and limit setting in which a parent engages. Imagine, here, a vertical axis, the *y*-axis in the figure. At the extreme bottom end of this continuum, parents apply virtually no limits at all—the child is essentially left to mature on her own. As the scale goes up, so does the parent's sense of being a clear authority figure, with use of regular expectations and demands for behavioral control and compliance. At the very top, parental authority is absolute, with a fully regimented structure.

Again, pause to assess where you might fall on this spectrum. Do you subscribe to the philosophy that too much structure might stifle your child's spontaneity and creativity? You might also be relatively low on this dimension if you would actually like to be more in control but are afraid of your child's responses—or her possible rejection of you if you imposed stronger limits. If you're on the top part of the scale, maybe you were raised in a boot-camp manner and have come to believe that this is the safest and most direct way to guide your child: clear rules, no excuses, and clear consequences for misbehavior. Or perhaps a lapse in your limits led to an incident or lack of safety for your child, which you wish to never happen again. Or you fear for the potential dangers of adolescence, so that you have clamped down hard in terms of demands and control as time has gone on.

Of course, the older a child becomes, the more authority and control parents need to hand off to the youth. This may start with allowing a growing child to play outside and continue with allowing the child to walk to the store unattended, all the way to the adolescent issues of attending parties, dating, and the like. Still, parents vary enormously in terms of their relative placement on this dimension, regardless of the child's age.

Four Fundamental Styles

Across the large amounts of research on these two dimensions, the usual finding is that they are unassociated. In other words, a parent's score on the first dimension (responsiveness/warmth) is essentially unrelated to that parent's score on the other dimension (control/demandingness). In practical terms, this means that parents who are quite similar on warmth/responsiveness may vary dramatically on authority/demandingness—and vice versa.

So, as you consider the figure once again, you'll see that the two dimensions are, in fact, at right angles to each other. That is, there are just about as many parents in the upper right quadrant (high on both dimensions) as there are in the other three quadrants. Even more, fascinating patterns emerge when we consider the kinds of parenting—and potential effects on their child—at the intersections of these two dimensions. Following is information on the four classic styles of parenting that emerge when responsiveness/warmth and control/demandingness are considered together.

Authoritative Parenting

Here, in the upper right part of the figure, a parent is higher than average on both dimensions, a pattern often termed *authoritative* or *authoritative/responsive*. This style comprises a real blend of the joy and acceptance related to the responsiveness/warmth dimension and the use of structure and limits related to the control/demandingness dimension. In short, parents are clearly happy in their parenting role and overtly warm with their offspring, but at the same time, they are not afraid to set clear limits and stick to them as much as possible.

> *Authoritative parenting is marked by a "firm, yet affirmative" set of parenting practices.*

As indicated by some of the adjectives in the figure, parents are both assertive and flexible. They are more than fine with setting limits, but—importantly—they explain those limits to the child during calm conversations that are removed from the time of any infractions. In other words, the relatively high demands and control are balanced by a democratic stance, through which the child comes to understand and learn the value of the limits. The parents set the rules, but, over the course of development, the child is a growing part of those negotiations.

Many scientists and child professionals consider such authoritative parenting to represent the ideal, in that its blend of noticeable limits plus real warmth and responsiveness presents a balanced backdrop against which the child can thrive academically and socially. According to this view, such a parenting style promotes self-regulation in the offspring, which can be particularly significant to your daughter with ADHD.

Here are a few other aspects of this parenting style that can be important in raising a daughter with ADHD:

• *Parents high on authoritative parenting tend to push their offspring toward independence and autonomy at age-expected times.* If they base this judgment on astute observations of their child, which tell them that the child is ready, the child can benefit (especially because kids with ADHD may be several years behind their peers in overall maturation, as noted in Chapter 4). A permissive parent (see below) may let the child or teen decide when it's time to move up the ladder toward independence, which could be disastrous for a girl with ADHD, who is vulnerable to poor self-regulation. Authoritarian parents (described in more detail below) may actually slow the child's independence because they tend to make most of the decisions about expectations for their offspring's behavior. This style could rob a girl with ADHD of the extra support in developing self-regulation that she needs.

• *Authoritative parents use negotiation and reasoning, rather than top-down commands (authoritarian) or the hope that the child will "see the light" (permissive).* That's why the term *democratic* is often used for parents who exemplify an authoritative style. This stance may be really important for kids with ADHD, who often lack the self-regulation to control their behavior on their own but may rebel against seemingly arbitrary parental control. Engaging them in reasoning about house rules can help to "bring them on board."

• *Parents in this quadrant tend to have clear, definite views on child rearing—but not so definitive that they omit their offspring from key aspects of family decision making.* As just noted, the deficits in executive function that come with ADHD leave girls with difficulty making good decisions and with planning and problem solving. Learning these important functions in the safety of the family can give them a boost.

As useful as authoritative parenting can be, there are also a couple of caveats to keep in mind:

• *Some children, particularly those with good self-control and reasonably stable and easy temperaments, may be easier to parent authoritatively than others.* This means that no matter how advantageous this parenting style may be to your daughter with ADHD, you may find it more challenging to be authoritative with her than it was with her siblings without ADHD. Once again, the age-old chicken-and-egg question: Do parents mold their children, or do child behavioral tendencies mold their parent's approach to them? The correct answer is "both of the above," as parent–child interactions are reciprocal and cyclic rather than unidirectional.

- *Any parent might not always be authoritative (or authoritarian, permissive, or uninvolved) and in the same ways for all children in a family.* As anyone who has grown up with one or more siblings knows, parents clearly have different attitudes and expectations for different kids in the same family. So, whereas there may be some truth in assuming a parent's general style is the same for all the children in the family, part of parenting is child-specific. In fact, research shows that the contextual factors that affect siblings *differently* (such as peers and child-specific parenting practices) have more bearing on later-life outcomes than those factors that affect all siblings in the same way (such as social class and general parenting styles). In short, you may need to adapt authoritative principles of parenting to your daughter with ADHD (for example, being gentler regarding some rules that are harder for her to remember but stricter on ones that might lead to danger if not followed consistently).

Authoritarian Parenting

In this (upper left) portion of the figure, the parent is high on control and demandingness but relatively lower on responsiveness and warmth. Here, there are benefits of limits but without the potential benefits of the warmth and connection of a more authoritative parenting style. This is a pattern in which parental directives hold the day. Primary here are rules, which must be followed; structure, which does not allow much in the way of deviation from such parental control; and high value placed on the child's obedience to such rules. Punishment is a key motivator. Again, these attitudes and practices are not balanced by the more democratic stance of the authoritative parent.

On average, children growing up in homes marked by a strongly authoritarian parenting style may emerge as fairly compliant and rule following. Or, depending on their temperamental styles or the influence of many other factors, they may become defiant and rebellious, in the hope of defying or breaking down such rules. But there are few absolutes here. Some ethnic groups and cultures place a priority on control/demandingness, whereas others may favor a more democratic style of child rearing. What's optimal in modern, 21st-century

America may be less adaptive elsewhere. And many children with ADHD may recoil against a strict authoritarian parental style that's not balanced by lots of warmth and support. In all, there are many factors that work together in shaping a child's ultimate outcomes.

Permissive Parenting

Here we flip to the bottom-right quadrant. The parent is above average on responsiveness and warmth but relatively lower (all the way to far lower) on control and limit setting. The priority here may well be on letting the child express herself, without dragging her down into social conformity. Her authentic self-expression may well be the parent's objective. Or, in other cases, the parent just doesn't assert much control.

In a home dominated by this parenting style, the child will typically "call the shots" more often than does the parent. At one level, the parent may be encouraging her creativity and expression, so she can flourish. Yet at another, the parent may not appreciate the dangers of letting the child be in control as much as she is. Even more, the parent may be fearful of the child's pushback if limits are set. Both of these issues may be relevant for a girl with ADHD, who could lack the intrinsic motivation and self-control to keep herself on track and motivated without strong support and control. Nonetheless, the parent's warmth and acceptance, along with responsiveness to the child's needs, are still felt.

On average (but remember, there is truly no average when it comes to parenting and child development), children of permissive parents may, if they possess good self-regulation and curiosity, thrive. On the other hand, if the child is lacking in such qualities and if the parent veers toward appeasement at all costs, even overindulging the child, the result could be a youth with little in the way of rule following, a low ability to negotiate school or engage in reciprocal relationships, or an inflated sense of self. Again, these outcomes may be particularly likely for some children with ADHD.

Uninvolved Parenting

Although there are few absolutes from the science of parenting, given huge differences across families and cultures, one is quite clear: The worst child outcomes emerge from parents in the uninvolved (all the way to neglectful) quadrant, at the lower left.

Here the parent is low on both responsiveness/warmth and control/ demandingness. For reasons of poor attachment from the parent's own past, poverty, substance abuse, or being overwhelmed by life stress, the caregiver is neither fundamentally interested/invested in the offspring's well-being nor able to provide more than rudimentary limits and controls on the child—at its extreme, to the point of neglect. Recall from Chapter 4 that extreme depriva- tion in early development can lead to high levels of inattention and overactiv- ity (along with attachment patterns linked to indiscriminate friendliness and other signs of extremely poor parent–child bonds). It may be the case that if you're fostering, or have adopted, a girl with ADHD who spent early years in a neglectful environment, it would be helpful to understand some of the potential impacts on her (see Resources, under "Trauma-Informed Care").

Which Style Is "Best" for a Child with ADHD?

As indicated, clearly there's a worst style—for a child with ADHD or for any child: the uninvolved quadrant, especially when it is severe enough to involve neglect. Otherwise, debate continues. Many scientists and clinicians believe that authoritative parenting most often predicts optimal outcomes, both aca- demically and socially. It's an intuitively appealing belief, in that the combi- nation of warmth and structure does appear optimal for child development. Across many research samples, this in fact does seem to be the case: Kids with authoritative parents do the best, on average, in school and in peer relation- ships.

But it's not that simple. Recall from Chapter 4 that it's difficult, if not impossible, to disentangle genes and environment where parenting is con- cerned. A parent and their biological child share half of their genes, and those genes shape both the parent's and the child's behavior. So it's hard to tell whether it's the parenting environment—such as authoritative or other parent- ing style—that really matters versus the genetic similarity between parent and child. This is especially true considering that children are inevitably shaped by parenting *and* that parents alter their parenting style in accord with the child's temperament or early behavior.

Given these complications, how do we figure out what parenting style is best for children with ADHD? The best test would be a completely unethical experiment of randomly assigning young children with (or at high risk for) ADHD to live with parents displaying markedly different parenting styles, for a decade or more, and then examining their long-term outcomes. As an alternative, my own lab attempted to address this question by having a group of carefully diagnosed boys with ADHD and a group of typically developing boys participate in summer camps where they could be observed in a natural setting.

Summer Camp Study of Boys with ADHD versus Boys without ADHD

In our study, the children rated one another in terms of social competence throughout the program. Prior to the camps, we also appraised parents with respect to their parenting styles. The objective was to observe which parenting style would predict which boys with ADHD would get the highest ratings for social competence from their peers (in terms of popularity and acceptance).

Authoritarian and permissive styles were reported about equally between the parents of boys with ADHD and the parents of the other boys. Yet the primary-caregiver parents (usually mothers) had far lower scores on the authoritative factor. Let's face it: Boys (and girls) with ADHD are not the easiest kids to parent. Such parents often report that good will has evaporated after years of struggles over rules and homework—and that, from fear over the child's noncompliance and rebellion, they have stopped enforcing many house rules. Even more, many such parents have given up on pushing their offspring to be autonomous, instead supporting them via "overhelp" or other means of avoiding conflict. Still, in this study, some of the caregivers of the boys with ADHD reported authoritative beliefs and practices that were just as strong as those of the highest scores of the comparison group's parents. In other words, it's still possible to maintain an authoritative parenting style even when raising an offspring with ADHD.

In this study, we used a number of variables to predict each boy's end-of-camp social appraisals by his peers, including daily observations of his behavior patterns from classroom and playground settings, parental history of mental disorder, and the primary parent's authoritative parenting score. To our surprise, we discovered that, for the ADHD sample, the key predictor of the boy's social competence was indeed

Authoritative parenting turns out to be important to the social competence of boys with ADHD—much more so than for boys without ADHD.

his caregiver's score on authoritative parenting. On the other hand, for the comparison group, this authoritative parenting score didn't really matter at all.

In short, our team revealed that an authoritative style blending warmth/ attachment *and* holding to clear limits—in other words, maintaining a *firm yet affirming parenting style,* as highlighted above—was associated with real benefits for kids with ADHD. It is no easy task for parents of youth with ADHD to maintain this style, but I believe that it is an essential goal. On the other hand, for the comparison group, authoritative parenting didn't really matter much with respect to competence with peers.

Think of it this way: There may well be many roots of socially competent behavior for a child without the challenges of ADHD. It might just "come naturally" to him or her. But for those with the diagnosis, promoting socially competent behaviors may take extra efforts on the part of families (and teachers). For such kids, the kind of parenting that is at once validating and supportive *plus* appropriately controlling may facilitate better social behavior.

Recall the orchid and dandelion metaphor from Chapter 4: If they receive extraordinary support from families, schools, and communities, those youth with genetic vulnerability to ADHD may well thrive in unexpected ways.

Studies of Adopted Boys and Girls

But wait: Our study involved boys only. And most of the families were biological in nature, so it was impossible to separate effects of shared genes from shared child-rearing experiences. Yet colleagues in England, led by Gordon Harold in the United Kingdom, have provided incredible evidence of the power of positive parenting for boys *and* girls with ADHD. Their research features the use of large samples of adoptive children—a huge step, because in adoptive families parents and children do not share common genes, allowing better separation of genetic from parenting influences.

> Research has shown that, even in a condition as biologically based as ADHD, parenting does matter, especially when the parenting involves warmth and structure rather than antagonism or an overly passive approach.

A series of important studies produced equally important findings:

- The *biological* mother's level of ADHD predicted the child's ADHD symptoms—even though the child had been adopted at birth, thus revealing the heritable nature of ADHD behaviors.

- Those early-childhood ADHD symptoms predicted the *adoptive* mother's levels of parental hostility, revealing that ADHD can elicit harsh parenting, even when there's no genetic connection between parent and child.

- The *adoptive* mother's hostility predicted continuing levels of ADHD symptoms across development (showing that parenting does matter, beyond genes).

Girls Only: What the BGALS Revealed about Parenting

But what about girls with ADHD exclusively? Our own research from the BGALS project has uncovered two critical findings:

1. *The key variable in predicting later negative outcomes was the level of the primary caregiver's stress and uncertainty about parenting.* Noteworthy problems in school and in self-control are not typical for girls to display. So, when they appear because of ADHD, they place a great deal of stress on the family (and, I believe, actively promote tendencies for self-blame in parents). Such parenting stress—which involves feeling overwhelmed and inadequate as a parent and questioning the closeness of the interactions with one's daughter—is a predictor of the daughter's key impairments in later life. Anything we as clinicians and researchers can do to bolster parenting confidence and competence—and to lower parenting stress—could go a long way toward preventing the kinds of negative outcomes too often in store for girls with ADHD as they grow out of childhood.

2. *A girl's report of negative interchanges with her father (but not with her mother) predicted engagement in later self-harm.* This came out of a relatively recent study published by our lab, which certainly needs to be confirmed by other labs. But these findings are reminiscent of other studies highlighting the importance of fathers for girls' development. Close bonds with a father (or father figure) may well protect girls with ADHD, in particular, against engagement in self-punishment and self-injury.

Other Parenting Practices

Research has shown that parenting practices and parental stress are not the only factors that matter to outcomes for girls with ADHD. The following three additional parenting behaviors and attitudes could really matter for you and your daughter.

Monitoring and Setting Limits

It's 11:00 P.M.: Where is your teenage daughter? This sentence captures one aspect of the important parental task of monitoring the whereabouts of a girl with ADHD.

Close monitoring is of course central to the very survival of any infant or young child. As your daughter matures, you need to promote greater independence, gradually, yet still with support and a clear sense of where she is and whether she's safe. By later childhood, early adolescence, and later adolescence, sensitive monitoring becomes extremely important.

For girls (and boys) heading toward and proceeding through puberty, the desire for independence, the clamoring for contact with peers, and the increasing desire to keep distance from one's parents are some of the most contentious sources of strife in family life. After all, the evolutionary "goal" of adolescence is attaining independence from one's family of origin, procreating, and beginning the process anew. Of course, we now live in an information-based world of ever-earlier puberty paired with ever-lengthier adolescence and emerging adulthood. Little wonder that tension, arguments, and threats are rampant.

Low parental monitoring is, not surprisingly, associated with risk for associating with peers who engage in risky behavior, including substance use/abuse and delinquency. Keeping tabs on one's children and thus being able to respond to trouble are crucial. Yet a major challenge for all families of youth this age is finding the right balance between protection and overprotection and between growing independence and "too much rope."

All these issues are especially loaded if your daughter has ADHD, with or without additional behavioral and emotional issues. As emphasized repeatedly, she may well be delayed in her neural development and self-regulation. Her impulsivity and fragile sense of self-worth may push her toward connection with peers who can provide temporary, albeit risky, support. More will follow on this topic in later chapters, but for now, I ask you to be aware of any tendency

> *Monitoring a daughter with ADHD is essential— but it's not likely to be effective without a strong parent–child bond.*

you may have toward looser versus tighter monitoring of your daughter as she grows up. Please consider thinking through your stance, while also remembering that appropriate monitoring is greatly facilitated by a strong bond between parent and child.

Striving for Consistency

Consistency in parenting can take place within a given parent over time and between two or more parents/caregivers who co-parent a particular girl.

Both are important. Let's face it: If your daughter hears you make a promise of a reward for something special that she does and you fail to deliver on it, her trust in you erodes. And if you say there will be a penalty for some misbehavior, such as failing to complete a set amount of homework or coming home too late—but don't follow through—she learns that she can get away with such rule breaking. This pattern fuels escalations of noncompliance, along with subsequent arguing and screaming bouts at home—which benefit no one. It's indeed hard to be consistent with your daughter with ADHD, but striving toward consistency should be a major objective.

Similarly, if parent number one is tough in terms of limits for the daughter but parent number two makes excuses and covers for her, guess which one she will turn to next time something is under dispute?

Clearly, these points look obvious on the written page—yet it's much harder to be consistent in the real world. Being a parent (and especially the parent of a girl with ADHD, who frankly requires more consistency than most other girls) mandates soul searching, a degree of toughness, and sheer effort to follow through on your limits and consequences. And, if you're co-parenting, it necessitates regular communication with your partner, lest one of you becomes the duped "easy mark" and the other the despised "bad cop." Consistent, high-quality parenting 24/7 is an unreachable dream, but your daughter with ADHD will benefit greatly the more you strive toward this ideal.

> *Consistency can close loopholes in rules and also avoid the dreaded "divide and conquer" tactic that teens might try in two-parent families.*

Creating a Fit

The notion of "fit" has to do with flexibility and adaptability in a parent–child relationship, particularly on the part of the parent. No child can ever attain the ideal that parents might have held for her as they anticipated her arrival into the world and their home. In particular, if an infant is intense when parents might have hoped for one with a calmer temperament, they will come to realize, sooner or later, that their ability to mold and shape this temperament has real limits. As another example, some parents might not quite understand an overly placid baby when they themselves are quite vigorous.

So, beyond the parenting practices and styles under discussion in this chapter, it's crucial that we as parents come to modify our own desires and tendencies—and appreciate our daughters' differences, creating the kind of "space" in the family where she fits. An overused metaphor here is that it's really hard, and typically quite unproductive, to fight fire with fire. But accepting differences, gradually building skills and competencies, and relishing your daughter's growth in ways that you might not initially have expected, can all be of huge benefit.

> *Finding a fit with the wider world can already feel like a challenge for your daughter with ADHD. Give her a good start by making sure she finds a fit at home.*

What Matters Most for a Girl with ADHD?

If you look beneath and beyond your daughter's surface behaviors, the ones stressing you out, you'll probably see signs of her acute awareness of how often she falls short in the eyes of many people in her world. She almost certainly won't tell you how astutely she perceives the disappointment in your eyes, her poor performance at school, her teachers' mistrust that she's really trying, or her classmates' belief that she may probably be just, well, weird. Still, you might sense her self-doubt. You might notice signs of shame—which she conveys through self-denigration or anger about your limit setting—that she has failed you and herself. Such signs might include lowered eyes or doubts that she can ever repair herself enough to truly live up to your standards. These signs are often subtle, but they often serve to drive you and her into different corners.

In such cases, your daughter merits understanding and support rather than additional blame and criticism, along with a commitment from you to facilitate the skills she needs to develop in terms of self-regulation, organization, and impulse control. This endeavor starts with adopting a parenting style that tries to eliminate bickering and arguing—and follows through on demands and promises. It continues with both warmth and appropriate limits, along with the three parenting practices described above: monitoring her carefully, striving for consistency (over time for yourself and also between you and her other parent/caregiver, if there is one), and creating a "fit" for her. It also takes the realization that there are many different paths to a fulfilling future for girls like her. Finally, it includes the following tasks:

- Engaging and reengaging with your daughter and seeking out her strengths—in short, showing her your warmth and acceptance
- Encouraging her to take small steps of progress—and providing rewards for doing so
- Being consistent with limits—and not caving in—when things get rough
- Keeping as even an emotional keel as you can
- Advocating for her among people who don't have such understanding (like wary teachers or school administrators or even neighbors and some relatives)

In the following chapters, I describe intervention strategies you can use in your role as a responsive and appropriately directive authoritative parent.

SIX

Core Treatments
for ADHD in Childhood
and Adolescence

You now have an overview of what ADHD is and what it looks like in girls, the best means of assessing it, its long-range outlook, what you need to know about its causes, and key principles of parenting—especially the need for (1) overcoming self-blame while resolving to help your daughter thrive and (2) blending warmth and responsiveness with clear limit setting. So this chapter focuses on core information on treatments that are supported by sound research. These involve behavioral and cognitive-behavioral strategies along with medications. Note that information abounds on a wide range of additional treatment strategies, accessible on many websites and other venues, often via promotions and advertisements. Although some of these additional treatments may be worthwhile, a lot of such information is just hype, supported by testimonials rather than actual research trials. In the case of ADHD, along with too many other child and adolescent mental health conditions, it's truly a case of *caveat emptor* ("let the buyer beware"). Try not to be misled.

Once you understand the basics of the intervention strategies with the best chance of success, turn to Chapter 7 for critical information on the crucial issue of educating your daughter with ADHD. I hasten to point out that it's not really possible to separate family and school in terms of interventions for girls with ADHD (or boys, for that matter). Still, there's so much important information here that the division into two chapters should make things clearer. Next, I emphasize which treatments, approaches, family supports, and educational plans work best for preschool- and grade-school-age girls (Chapter 8) and then for teens (Chapter 9). Although basic principles of treatment are similar for both age groups, there are enough differences between 7-year-old and 16-year-old

girls—and how treatments look and work for students in grade-school versus high-school—that separating the information into two chapters makes the
information most useful in a practical way. Finally, in Chapter 10 I synthesize
the book's essential messages and help you look forward to your daughter's
emergence into adulthood.

Before delving into treatments, consider whether you have worked through
the range of reactions and emotions that you might have had to your daughter's
diagnosis with ADHD. As I noted at the end of Chapter 2, these reactions might
include denial, grief, confusion, or even gratitude that you know what is causing
your daughter to struggle, that it's not your fault, and that now you can begin to
address it. A key advantage of the group-based behavioral family therapy discussed in this chapter is the chance to understand the kinds of reactions and
responses that other parents and families are having, even though the main
focus of this treatment is working on behavior change in yourself and your
daughter. It will also help to voice your reactions to your clinician (or clinicians,
if both medication and educational supports are also part of the treatment plan),
so that they can understand that simply diving into treatment may well take
some adjustment and processing at first. You may also be worried about the
stigma that often comes with a mental health diagnosis like ADHD. I hope the
knowledge you've gained in Chapters 3–5 has brought you to the realization that
a diagnosis can be far more than a source of
stigma. In fact, it may be the motivator to begin
the treatment process with a positive outlook.

*Working through your
emotional reactions
to your daughter's
diagnosis can be the
kick-start to effective
treatment.*

You should also be aware that amid the
often bewildering menu of treatments commonly touted as beneficial for ADHD, there
are only two fully evidence-based approaches
for such youth, supported by large numbers of
carefully controlled research studies:

1. *Behavioral approaches,* especially those that aim to teach you how to
   motivate and discipline your child more effectively while increasing
   positive family interactions (and involving coordination with parallel
   school-based efforts)—along with *cognitive-behavioral strategies* for
   teens and adults

2. *Medications,* usually the class called *stimulants*—a confusing name,
   which I'll explain—but also including other kinds of meds

Behavioral treatments (and their counterpart cognitive-behavioral treatments for older teens and adults) are based on the idea that the more regular, the more positive and reward-heavy, and the more consistent the environment is for a girl (or boy) with ADHD, the better the odds that she will develop self-regulation and academic/social skills. Medications for ADHD involve boosting the functioning of the neurotransmitter dopamine, as well as its counterpart norepinephrine, to promote better attention, self-regulation, and intrinsic motivation. As highlighted below, research reveals that it is typically a combination of the right kind and right dose of medication *and* a coordinated home/school behavioral program that has the best chance of helping your daughter with ADHD function at her very best. Once more, it's not biology *or* context but instead both, acting in concert, that usually provide the best means of making a real difference in behavior and life functioning.

Behavioral and Cognitive-Behavioral Treatments

As noted earlier, most treatments for ADHD—especially when it's evident in childhood and early adolescence—do not involve individual psychotherapy between the youth and a therapist. Instead, behavioral and cognitive-behavioral treatments emphasize modifying home and school environments to shape better functioning. Sometimes, though, if there's substantial trauma involved in her background, the child or teen may well benefit greatly from one-on-one therapy or counseling in order to work through the core idea that what happened to her was not her fault. The same is true for comorbid depression or serious anxiety: Individual (or group) cognitive-behavioral therapy, or another variety called *interpersonal therapy,* can provide real help. But if the main goal is to improve the core symptoms of ADHD, along with the many related impairments that accompany it (social issues, academic problems, discordant family interactions), the core approach is to create a more positive and structured environment at home and at school. It takes active involvement of the adults in a girl's environment to promote such skill building. Over time, the aim is for her to internalize the gains and positive feedback through finding ways to cope with and adapt to her ADHD-related issues, while obtaining the means to translate them into a productive life. Cognitive-behavioral therapy can provide just such skills in adolescence and beyond.

Let's dig a bit deeper. What works best for people with ADHD is not so much focusing on deep awareness of their early childhood but instead providing the optimal means of supporting skill development, largely from alterations in expectations and rewards delivered by parents and teachers. Included here is promoting better organizational skills and social skills for your daughter. The term *behavioral* comes from theories of learning that spurred what used to be called "behavior modification": the use of rewards and prudent punishments to shape positive behavior change. But things have moved well beyond M&M's (the stereotypic rewards in old-school "behavior mod"). In fact, through cognitive-behavioral therapy, as she gets older, your daughter becomes engaged in working on her own self-management and reward programs.

Behavioral Family Therapy (Parent Management Training)

There are a number of validated behavioral family approaches to reducing problem behavior and increasing motivation in children and teens with ADHD. Note that many of these are also applicable to youth with aggressive behavior patterns. The Resources section at the back of the book lists such programs. My aim here is to emphasize their similarities rather than highlight their particular differences. In some cases, parents work individually with a behavioral therapist, focusing on their daughter, whereas in other cases group intervention is provided. Ample evidence exists to support the effectiveness of both. Importantly, a group format allows parents to learn from and support one another. Moreover, this format can be supplemented, every few weeks, with the therapist's individual check-ins with a given family, to make sure that the principles and practices imparted to the group are applied specifically to the individual and family in question.

The general principles related to behavioral treatments correspond directly to the material in the initial chapters of the book. That is, given that kids with ADHD often have issues with slowed development of the prefrontal cortex of their brains and therefore show delays in self-regulation and self-management, as well as reduced intrinsic motivation, individual therapies attempting to foster emotional insight are usually barking up the wrong tree. Instead, the aim is to foster a better-regulated, highly positive, and encouraging set of situations at home and school, where your daughter can, slowly at first, gain skills and a growing sense that she can succeed. From there, family interactions should become less fraught, teachers can come to realize that your daughter is really trying, and a stronger sense of self-worth can emerge as your daughter encounters success.

But how can parents, especially those who may be prone to sharing some of the same characteristics as their offspring, create such an environment—and work with their daughter's teachers to foster the same kinds of structure and rewards? The short answer is that it takes commitment, dedication, resolve, and an emerging sense that change is possible. Required are (1) building a renewed sense of closeness to and attachment with your daughter, (2) working slowly but surely on skill development and rewards for such, and (3) maintaining a clear set of limits that can be enforced with firm yet nonemotional interactions.

To begin with, know that there are a large number of research investigations comparing behavioral family interventions to control conditions (for example, families who receive the sessions later) or to other, less behaviorally oriented, treatments. It's clear from such research that the chances of improvement in the child's behavior patterns are strong, as long as the family remains committed to change. Furthermore, when such behavioral family interventions include work with teachers (see Chapter 7), gains in school-related behavior and some key aspects of academic performance are evident as well.

Eight Principles of Behavioral Family Treatments

Despite some differences in emphasis and focus, most evidence-based parent/family behavioral treatments emphasize these principles:

1. Understanding more about ADHD

2. Rebonding with your daughter

3. Being specific in understanding (and monitoring) her behavior—both positive and negative aspects

4. Breaking down "target" behaviors into small steps

5. Applying what's called a functional analysis—that is, sequences of antecedent → behavior → consequence that can promote measurable change

6. Providing frequent, contingent, and consistent rewards for your daughter's skill building

7. Learning to apply judicious and nonemotional consequences for pre-agreed-upon negative behaviors

8. Rewarding yourselves as parents for all this effort, gradually fading rewards, and planning for the application of these behavioral principles outside the home setting

The following sequence often applies.

1. *Understanding ADHD.* First you'll learn important concepts about ADHD, a process formally called *psychoeducation.* The information here involves the kinds of points made in the initial chapters of this book on the nature of ADHD, its causes, and the importance of considering both biology and experience to move forward. The goal is to foster empathy and respect while reducing self-blame.

2. *Rebonding.* Next, many programs will promote a more positive attachment, or bond, between you and your daughter before moving on to specific behavioral principles and practices. For all the reasons noted in Chapter 5 related to attachment, this is really important. One way of doing this is to have you perform an exercise with your daughter regularly for a week or two. Here you allow your daughter to lead an activity—and you are not allowed to ask questions or direct it but instead can comment on her narrative during your time together (perhaps a favorite hobby of hers, anything that she enjoys). In my experience, many parents directly question the need for this exercise: "She's failing a class at school and has refused to do chores for weeks on end, but you're asking me to simply talk with her and reflect on her interests? Come on! We need to get serious here!" But it's often incredible how the same parents, a short time later, will come back to the group or individual session and remark on how great it is to connect with their daughter in a stress-free way. This process cannot, of course, overturn a long history of seriously disrupted bonding, but it can, in many cases, help you and your daughter reconnect in positive ways, an essential goal if you are to begin to be the source of clearer, meaningful limits and the dispensing of rewards for academic and behavioral progress.

3. *Getting specific about behaviors and recording your daughter's behaviors.* Next, you work on becoming more *specific* in observations of your daughter's performance, as well as your own patterns of interaction with your daughter.

In behavioral approaches—which emphasize modeling desirable behavior and providing rewards for small steps toward improvement—you learn to replace such global terms as "bad attitude," "stubbornness," "forgetfulness," or "spaciness" with specific observations, such as the following:

- Getting up from the dinner table too early (count the minutes!)
- Abandoning homework after frustration (how many problems attempted and completed correctly?)
- Failing to get ready for school in the frantic moments before your daughter has to leave the house (how many times was the school bus missed last week?)
- Seeming not to listen when you give directions (how often did you have to repeat the request?).

If you persist in bemoaning your daughter's global shortcomings, it's impossible to know which specific behaviors to target for intervention—and also impossible to know when improvement is actually taking place. At the same time, documenting specific behaviors eliminates the kind of character assassination that can creep into the picture via overly general attributions and criticism.

At the same time, you learn to keep actual records of your daughter's behavior. Again, the aim is to prevent the overly global and overly negative views of her performance that tend to develop. When you write or chart just what she actually does during the morning routine, mealtimes, homework sessions, or family outings, you are less likely to characterize her as generally lazy or defiant, thereby motivating work on specific behaviors. By measuring, you and your daughter can notice change more readily than if your observations constitute an overly global "all versus none" depiction. Crucially, the record-keeping serves as the basis for rewards (see step 6 below).

4. *Taking small steps.* Here you work on discovering the specific, small steps through which your daughter can build skills. Rome wasn't built in a day—or, to use another familiar phrase, a journey of a thousand miles begins with a single step. Expecting behavior change to accelerate from zero to 100 in a few seconds or minutes (or even a few days) is expecting too much from anyone, much less a girl with ADHD. It's a setup for failure. Start slowly and go from there. For example, if your daughter is currently sitting for 5 minutes at dinner before getting up without being excused, make the initial target a couple

of minutes longer—and then gradually work up from there, rather than insisting on a full mealtime at the start.

5. *Building the crucial skill of understanding the ABCs of the behavioral approach.* Specifically, this process of "functional analysis" involves determining the **A**ntecedents (conditions, expectations, requests) that can lead to certain **B**ehaviors (again measured specifically rather than globally), which are then followed by **C**onsequences that either increase or decrease the likelihood of the behavior's continuation. For example, an unclear or overly complex set of directions may lead to lack of follow-through or erratic performance by your daughter. Criticizing your daughter for this may increase her frustration and make her less likely to listen in the future. This analysis strongly suggests (1) altering the antecedents, by giving clear and simple directions—and then, when your daughter complies with your instructions, (2) responding with praise rather than criticism. In a different example, if you request quick completion of all homework (the antecedent) but your daughter stalls or refuses to perform (the problem behavior)—and you let her get away with nonperformance (wrong consequence)—she is likely to learn that delay and noncompliance provide "gains" for her refusal. Here a smaller "load" of homework (better antecedent) should produce greater completion and the consequence of a mark or star on her reward chart.

With the behavioral approach, you mold your own commands and directions—even through arranging the physical space in the home (so as to discourage doing homework in the living room in front of the TV)—to encourage success. Then follow your daughter's positive behavior, measured specifically, with rewarding consequences (praise, points on a chart that can be traded for desired goods or activities) and her negative behaviors with undesired consequences (loss of points, time-out for serious misbehavior). Once again, the goal is not deep understanding of longstanding family interactions or personal histories but instead a far more direct approach to encouraging and rewarding positive behavior and enforcing prudent negative consequences for problem behavior.

6. *Providing rewards.* You will learn to provide rewards for your daughter's initially small steps and then larger gains. As described earlier, those with ADHD do not naturally or easily develop intrinsic motivation. Slower brain development, along with aberrations in the flow of the neurotransmitter dopamine through crucial brain circuits, render them dependent on external signs and motivators. Reward charts map targeted skills to be developed and crucial

problem behaviors to be reduced onto simple graphs or figures, with rewards provided regularly for success. The goal, here, is positive interactions. Small units of behavior will earn small rewards (genuine praise and encouragement; one checkmark on a reward chart). And larger numbers of checks or stars on the chart will culminate in larger rewards over time. As noted in Chapters 8 and 9, incentive programs will look considerably different for a teenage girl with ADHD than for a first- or second-grader.

It's essential to remember that the reward to be given is an activity that your daughter really wants to do, not necessarily what you believe she should want to spend her time doing. This is why you need to engage her directly in the choice of rewards. It's always a good idea to have a range of rewards, as kids with ADHD are notorious for "satiating" on the same reward given over and over. Otherwise, even the best-planned behavioral charts can fail.

A few important tips for providing positive consequences and rewards: When your daughter is learning a new skill or attempting to reduce a problematic behavior, the more praise, encouragement, and reward points or stars that you can give, the better. In fact, rewards need to be given consistently and genuinely—and it's important to give praise or place the star on the refrigerator chart *only* when the behavioral goal in question is accomplished. Over time, though, you'll want to taper your rewards to a less regular, less predictable schedule, which will help ensure that your daughter's gains persist.

7. *Imposing negative consequences.* Once rewards are in place, some amount of noncompliant or disruptive behavior will inevitably exceed the clear limits that you've established. At those times, it's crucial that you enforce such limits via brief time-outs or subtractions of some of the points or stars your daughter has gained. All this should be laid out crisply and clearly ahead of time. Then, when an infraction occurs, there can be no bickering or negotiating related to these consequences—in fact, stalling and prolonged negotiations will send a message that your daughter can get away with almost anything and get plenty of attention for it! Furthermore, you must deliver the negative consequences without resorting to yelling, scolding, or castigating. In fact, the progression of such hostile interchanges, related to parental caving in, failing to follow through, and eventual sarcasm/bitterness, must be avoided at all costs. They are a clear step on the pathway from ADHD to more frankly aggressive or self-destructive behavior. Please see the box on the next page on the best ways to use negative consequences judiciously.

Tips for Effective Use of Negative Consequences

It would be awesome if treatment for ADHD involved only praise and rewards, but research clearly indicates that real limits—backed up by negative consequences, prudently and nonemotionally delivered—are also required. Here is some advice for making this part of a behavioral program work:

• Understand that the intent is not to be cruel but instead to protect your daughter, and the family's safety, and to deliver the message that positive behavior is expected, with real consequences if it is not forthcoming.

• Make sure rules/limits have been preestablished and discussed with your daughter and are not seat-of-the-pants rules made up at the height of your anger.

• When you have to deduct points or stars from her behavioral chart, make that subtraction clearly but without ridiculing or shaming her.

• Use time-out (on a chair, with no access to her toys or games) with a relatively young child. Prudent use of time-out does not disrupt attachment but instead fosters it.

• Refrain from, or at least take real care with, any actual physical punishment. This is a major issue these days in the United States, in different subcultures, and internationally. Is a spank on the rear end ever justified? Perhaps for a toddler who is on the verge of running into traffic . . . but rarely in older youth and never when the primary aim is to express the anger or outrage you may be experiencing. If ever justified, it must be done without negative emotion and with extreme consistency—otherwise, the child may become inured to pain. There is also the potential for abuse if physical punishment is used indiscriminately. This is why there are increasing calls never to use any physical punishment, ever.

• Don't let negative consequences outweigh rewards. Make sure there is a really high ratio of positive expectations, praise, and rewards to penalties and point subtractions. If you find your daughter in a "deficit economy"—such that she has a negative balance of points on her reward system—something is clearly wrong. Make sure at the beginning that there will be more points for incremental steps toward positive behavior than penalties for negative behavior. A good aim is a 5:1 ratio (or even higher) of positive to negative comments. Otherwise, the whole reward program will backfire.

8. *Using self-rewards, fading, and applications outside the home.* Throughout this work, you need to reward *yourself* for the sometimes mundane but often challenging efforts involved in setting up the kind of behavioral programs and reward charts just described. Essential features here are focusing on one or two target goals at a time before moving to other goals, the rewarding of progress, and enforcement of negative consequences for clear violations without the pleading, begging, anger, and arguing that can seriously erode family harmony and spur ever-worsening interactions. Don't forget that doing all this requires real changes on your part, so remember to give yourself some "cred"!

Over time you will also learn how to gradually taper the rewards, once problem behaviors are under better control and skills are being built, so that your daughter can begin to display greater self-regulation and self-control. This last phase is not quick or easy—in fact, it can take a lifetime for any of us to become better regulated, and this challenge is extremely salient if your daughter has ADHD. Finally, although space does not allow detail here, you will also need to learn how (especially for younger kids) to apply the reward charts and occasional need for consequences like time-out on outings beyond the home.

Your Essential Role

As you consider what you will be doing during behavioral family therapy, don't underestimate the magnitude of the shift you will probably need to make so that this treatment is effective. You need to become a teacher, a guide, and a coach of your daughter's attempts to self-regulate. All this may very well mean getting a greater hold on your own emotions, gaining a greater understanding of your own guilt or shame (for example, that you believe you have caused all of your daughter's issues), and a deep transcending of your potential fear that you will disappoint or anger your daughter if you dare to set and hold to clear limits. Behavioral parent management of youth with ADHD is quite specific, in keeping with the behavioral perspective that the focus is on clear goals and objectives. But it also requires a kind of broad and wise perspective—namely, that you'll need to radically rethink the origins of your daughter's problematic attention and behaviors, as well as your own role in shaping a more positive future.

Although little research on behavioral parent therapy has focused specifically on girls with this condition, existing studies reveal that girls fare comparably to boys when parents get deeply involved in these procedures. I suspect, however, that the "ask" for parents of daughters with ADHD is not simple here. For one thing, stress in the parenting role is particularly high for families of girls with ADHD—partly because of the "less expected" nature of ADHD in girls, with resultant stigma from society along with self-blame and even shame for parents. Additionally, behavioral parent therapy originated in work on boys with oppositional and defiant issues, which often co-occur with ADHD in males. Yet girls are more likely to have the inattentive presentation of ADHD, so some behavioral programs might have to be modified to focus on issues pertaining to lack of focus and organization (see the box at the end of this chapter for information on the Child Life and Attention Skills program, one of several more specifically targeted behavioral programs available for kids with the inattentive form of ADHD). Even so, the dynamics of family interactions can be truly fraught when a daughter has ADHD, requiring both acceptance *and* motivation for change on the part of parents. Sound difficult? I believe that it is, indeed! Yet it's doable.

> *Your role in behavioral family therapy may be even more important than it is for parents of boys— and more difficult to enact.*

Does the information here remind you of what was stated in Chapter 5 about authoritative parenting? It should! The aims of behavioral parent management are indeed to foster a more positive, warm, and responsive set of family interactions while simultaneously upping the structure and limit setting necessary to motivate and guide your daughter. Despite the often-held stereotype that behavioral approaches to parenting are cold and mechanistic, they are actually far from it. Reasonable goals, the use of planning sessions with your daughter about the reward program, generous praise, and enforcement of house rules and limits without resorting to cajoling/arguing/yelling are all part of the master plan with respect to behaviorally oriented parent management. It's particularly important not to invalidate your daughter's experiences by somehow implying that her ADHD problems are simply the result of her not trying—or of intentional attempts to get back at you. Such messages of denying the reality of her experiences can have seriously negative consequences as she moves into adolescence and beyond.

Finally, from reading this material, you might come to believe that this approach can be performed by simply following the guidelines presented. But it's much more difficult to do all this than you might think. Above all, it takes practice—and clear guidance from the therapist who conducts the behavioral family intervention. In fact, much of the content of behavioral family treatments is enacted through role-plays and practice sessions (and sometimes video modeling), rather than lectures or book learning. Old habits can be hard to break, meaning that active modeling, guidance, and feedback are core elements for success. More specialized behavioral treatments are highlighted in the box on pages 146–147.

Note that a core aspect of behavioral parenting interventions is to get parents deeply involved in their daughter's school performance as well. Specifically, the same principles that apply to behavior management and skill development at home should be echoed at school by her teachers. As noted, I defer this part of behavioral interventions to Chapter 7, when I take up the whole topic of educating your daughter with ADHD. But remember, the best behavioral parenting interventions include directly reaching out to schools and teachers as a crucial part of the process of coordinating expectations between home and classroom.

Social Skills Training

As highlighted in earlier chapters, a large percentage of youth with ADHD experience difficulties with peers. Some—usually those who are impulsive and aggressive—are likely to be actively rejected by agemates, leading to a cascade of low self-esteem, loss of social contacts, and attraction to peers interested in rule-breaking behavior, substance abuse, and the like. Others, like those with inattentive-style ADHD, may be ignored more than actively rejected, perhaps because of a lack of positive social skills, including difficulties in reading social cues accurately. Thus, another behaviorally based intervention for this crucial target area is social skills training.

Briefly, the premise is that adults may not be the best teachers or coaches for advancing social skills. Instead, the optimal avenue is direct contact with other youth. Yet rather than the kinds of group therapy that promote expression of feelings, the behavioral social skills approach is far more directive and rehearsal oriented. Here, with a group of four to eight kids with ADHD, the therapists have a list of specific "targets" (for example, introducing oneself, taking turns, encouraging peers) that are modeled and practiced in a highly structured way. Ample rewards are provided not only for paying attention to the content of the group but for trying out and practicing the skills taught.

The evidence here is not as strong, however, as it is for behavioral family therapy and its variants. For one thing, there are fewer published reports on social skills training. For another, if the group sessions lack structure and order, some participants may model negative social behaviors that other participants may copy, resulting in worse behavior. In these cases, social skills interventions can backfire. Still, evidence exists that with well-trained and warm/structured leaders, more socially skilled behavior, and even friendships, can build. Above all, it's not just skill learning but skill practicing—under realistic group interactions—that's the active ingredient. A number of clinicians and advocates regarding ADHD believe that such social skills/group-based approaches are particularly helpful for girls with ADHD, though more research is needed to bear this belief out.

In another variation of social skills training, parents of younger girls (and boys) with ADHD are taught by therapists to facilitate playdates—often, for youth with ADHD, a rare occurrence in the real world—to provide the direct kinds of social learning required to build positive social interactions.

Cognitive-Behavioral Therapy

As children with ADHD become teenagers and then adults, it's logical to think (or at least hope) that they may be able to take charge of their own behavioral strategies and treatment plans. In fact, 50 years ago, the movement to promote behavioral/reward-based treatments for a range of psychological problems began to find common ground with "cognitive therapy," a form of psychological treatment that featured the direct targeting of people's thinking strategies. What has emerged is a strong, evidence-based range of treatments blending behavioral and cognitive strategies, called *cognitive-behavioral therapy (CBT)*.

For adults with depression, anxiety, or a range of other emotional issues, CBT targets the kinds of rigid and distorted thinking patterns that can amplify the symptoms at hand. For example, if I'm clinically depressed, I might think that I'm always a failure, that nothing I do can make a difference—and that any additional evidence of even small mistakes ("I said the wrong thing at work and everyone knew it") piles on and makes me feel even more helpless and hopeless. In CBT, the therapist challenges such negative thinking and asks me to try out other ways of construing the situation ("maybe I just goofed—and I'm not doomed forever"). I then actively check on my feeling states before and after trying out the alternative interpretation. Although this is a highly simplistic depiction, CBT has been found in hundreds of studies to help adults form a different picture of themselves and emerge from depression.

But when such cognitive strategies have been tried with kids experiencing ADHD, the concepts don't readily "take." Perhaps the slower cognitive and emotional development of these youth requires a more basic, reward-based, behavioral approach. For older teens and adults with ADHD, however, CBT makes use of the behavioral principles of positive and negative consequences to foster self-control and self-regulation, actively applied to longstanding cognitive, behavioral, and emotional patterns. In fact, a growing number of studies reveals that, for this age group, a CBT approach that emphasizes self-monitoring, self-reward, organizational skills, time management, and anger control can produce real change. CBT for ADHD is not available everywhere, so be on the lookout in your area.

Medication

Medications for ADHD, particularly the class called *stimulants,* have been around longer than modern psychotropic medication for other mental and neurodevelopmental disorders. They were first demonstrated to be helpful for youth with ADHD-like behavior patterns in the late 1930s, although it took 20-plus more years before they became widely used. Despite their long history, these medications remain controversial for several reasons:

• Many people believe that it's unethical to medicate youth with low self-regulation or other ADHD-related issues, which should instead be treated psychosocially. Most professionals, however, from appraising the large numbers of relevant research studies, know that benefits can be quite positive.

• In the general population, the potential for addiction to stimulant medications is real. Although for children with ADHD there is extremely low potential for such, for teens and adults, the chances rise—meaning that doctors and families must closely monitor the medications prescribed. And, as noted below, when non-ADHD teens and adults take stimulants to boost performance, there is a real chance for addiction to develop (all the more reason to keep close tabs).

• Pills cannot, in and of themselves, create positive academic and social skills. Still, in many cases medications can facilitate better learning for individuals with ADHD when paired with good academic and behavioral programs.

• A common belief is that the pharmaceutical industry has profited far too much from medicalizing and medicating a number of problems in functioning that are actually not mental disorders. This view can lead to blanket assertions that stimulants are agents of "mind control" for ADHD. But the science behind the benefits of stimulants is strong.

How Should You Make Decisions about Medications for Your Daughter?

It would take a lot more space than is available here to address all these points thoroughly. But here are some initial thoughts.

First, let's (wrongly) assert the belief that ADHD has no biological basis and that genes have no bearing on its symptoms. If so, perhaps medications actually are an attempt to change brains illegitimately, even unethically. Yet biological roots can be real. Should we urge that nearsighted or farsighted individuals forgo glasses or contact lenses and just "try harder"? Or that people with cancer should "will away" the cancerous cells? Both ideas are incredibly insensitive, stigmatizing, and just wrong. Yet many still don't quite "get" that ADHD (especially in girls) is a lot more than a lack of effort.

Second, all treatments—whether psychosocial or medical—have potential side effects, which must be balanced against positive effects. Medications for ADHD are no different, but the issues become particularly loaded when it's believed that medicating inattentive or impulsive behavior is unethical or even immoral. Note that chemotherapy for cancer has noteworthy side effects, as do medications for any other biomedical condition. In the case of stimulants, the potential for addiction is real, as noted above and discussed below, if the medications are in the wrong hands. But what's required is a real reconciliation of the facts that (1) these medications are highly established as effective (at least in the short term) while (2) any benefits must be weighed in light of the costs for a particular individual.

Third, as highlighted below, medications may be essential for some individuals with ADHD, and quite helpful for others. But except in rare cases—in which the individual in question has mild to moderate ADHD with no additional conditions—pills alone cannot be the entire treatment regimen. Family interactions, teacher–student interactions, and altered sense of self-worth must all be targeted as well, which is where combinations of behavioral and medication treatments are crucial.

Finally, "Big Pharma" has taken it on the chin, justifiably in many cases, for overpromoting and overselling medications. On the other hand, the government alone can never provide the levels of funding needed to develop new medication treatments for a range of conditions. What I believe we should do, crucially, is weigh the sins of the for-profit pharmaceutical industry against the benefit of medications that can save and improve lives. This is no easy journey in the world of ADHD, but a large number of objective studies have shown just how much ADHD-related medications can help.

It's a parent's job to be careful about authorizing medication or any other treatment, but remember that the most important factor to consider is how much the treatment is likely to help your daughter.

Stimulants

What are stimulants? It's a misleading name, for sure. Unless doses are too high or unless such medicines are used for abuse, stimulants for ADHD actually enhance focus and self-regulation by "stimulating" regulatory systems in the brain. At a biological level, this class of medications accentuates the actions of the neurotransmitter called *dopamine*. The pills block the reabsorption of dopamine, once it has been released into the synapse (the small gap between neurons), allowing the released dopamine to continue its actions on the next neuron in the pathway, making it fire electrically—and so on down the chain.

In this way, a better name for this type of medication would be *selective dopamine reuptake inhibitor (SDRI)*—parallel to the way many antidepressants are SSRIs, or selective serotonin reuptake inhibitors. (Actually, stimulants enhance the actions of both dopamine and norepinephrine, so that they should be called SDNRIs, but I'm now getting too complicated for our own good.) Because one of the primary neural pathways involving dopamine works to modulate alertness and attention, stimulants can definitely help with the core symptoms of ADHD. In fact, therapeutic doses of stimulant medications act to calm overactive behavior and enhance the focus of the individual in question, rather than "stimulate" her in the way you might envision from that term.

Here's how this works: When a girl with ADHD takes a stimulant dosage, about 20 minutes later, once the medicine is in the bloodstream and enters the brain, dopamine levels are increased. Thus, alertness goes up and distractibility goes down. Because there are also dopamine pathways deep inside the brain, related to motivation, formerly boring or uninteresting tasks now engender more interest and focus. Dopamine is also carried in a large brain circuit linking the prefrontal cortex with other brain regions, so that executive functions, especially inhibition, are enhanced. Overall, for those girls and boys with ADHD who show a positive response (about 80%, if the right type of stimulant and the right dosage are established for the particular individual), attention is boosted, impulsivity and extraneous motor behavior decrease, and the individual is temporarily more motivated. I say "temporarily" because stimulants don't last very long in the bloodstream or brain, ranging from 3–4 to 10–12 hours (depending on whether short- versus longer-acting formulations are prescribed), meaning that regular dosing each day is required.

Sometimes positive effects on ADHD symptoms appear the same morning of the first dose—and are quite noticeable. This is typically the case for highly impulsive and active individuals. In other cases, it takes a number of weeks to find the right kind of stimulant and the right dose (not too high, or side effects can emerge; not too low, or there's essentially no clinical benefit). This is more often the case for those with the inattentive presentation of ADHD. Side effects include suppression of appetite, wakefulness (a problem if doses are given too late in the day, preventing sleep), anxiety or compulsive/repetitious behavior, and (over the long haul) the potential for slowing physical growth (height) by about an inch. As with any medication, the balance of positive effects to side effects must be monitored and weighed carefully. In people without ADHD, especially teens and adults, stimulants can be addictive drugs of abuse. This is not usually the case for valid cases of ADHD, but close medical monitoring is needed.

In fact, doctors who prescribe ADHD medications should never simply write a prescription and assume that everything will subsequently be fine. For example, there is no blood test, or genetic examination, to determine who will respond best to the "methylphenidate" type of stimulants (like Ritalin, Concerta, or Focalin) versus the "amphetamine" type of stimulants (like Dexedrine, Adderall, or Vyvanse)—or at which dose. It therefore takes a careful, scientific, trial-and-error approach.

Although many individual differences exist, on average youth with the inattentive presentation of ADHD respond preferentially to lower doses of the medicine than those with more impulsive varieties (and, as highlighted earlier, girls are more likely than boys to display inattention as the predominant symptom). Thus, unless you work carefully with your doctor, there's a real chance that your daughter with ADHD could get overmedicated (and show side effects) right out of the gate, when a slower and more cautious approach might reveal medication benefits.

Please see the Resources at the back of the book for the link to an extremely useful medication guide that features most current ADHD medications.

Nonstimulants

The other main type of medicine that helps people with ADHD selectively acts on the neurotransmitter norepinephrine, enhancing its effects in one of several ways. Because these medications do not target dopamine directly, they do not give the clear "attentional boost" that stimulants are likely to foster. On the other hand, they lack the potential for dopamine-related side effects (though they come with their own set of side effects)—and they do not carry addiction potential. Instead, they tend to help more generally and slowly with impulse control and self-regulation.

One type of such medication is an SNRI (selective norepinephrine reuptake inhibitor). The most salient example is atomoxetine (Strattera). The other major type had been used to treat high blood pressure for some years before they were found to be effective for ADHD. They are sometimes therefore called "antihypertensive" medications or "alpha-2" medications (because they work on the alpha-2 receptors for norepinephrine). For a thorough review of medications for ADHD, both stimulants and nonstimulants, see, in the Further Reading section for this chapter, the citation of Chapter 9 of the 2022 book by Russell Barkley (*Treating ADHD in Children and Adolescents: What Every Clinician Needs to Know*), as well as the ADHD medication guide listed in the Resources at the back of the book.

Overall Benefits and Limitations

Hundreds of studies have compared the effects of ADHD-related medications to placebo pills, with outcome measures of parent- and teacher-rated behavior, objective observations, tests of cognitive performance, and key areas of life functioning. Some of these investigations span periods of hours or a few days, whereas others span a year or more. The overall conclusions may be surprising to you: Of all psychiatric medications for youth, the stimulants used for

ADHD have shown the strongest behavioral and cognitive effects, with the clear majority (70–90%) of youth with ADHD showing a positive response but far lower numbers showing a positive placebo response. The nonstimulant medicines for ADHD (studied mainly in the past couple of decades, with many fewer investigations) also yield effects that are well above placebo rates, though not, on average, as sizable as those for stimulants.

Beyond attention span or fidgeting, medication can help with the following:

- Aspects of school performance, even with respect to some academic tests

- Peer interactions (especially reducing negative responses from age-mates linked to improvements in an individual's impulsive behavior)

- Negative parent–child interactions (though medications do not, in and of themselves, do much to improve positive parenting behaviors—parents need to learn those from behavioral family therapy)

Medication's effects are sizable, on average, but usually not enough to place the child in the range of functioning of typical peers. As stated above, a combination of behavioral and medication treatments is most often needed for such gains.

Crucially, effects of medications usually don't persist once the medication is stopped. Performance is boosted as long as the active ingredients remain in the bloodstream and brain, but the effects aren't permanent. The holy grail for any intervention strategies related to ADHD, in fact, is whether benefits appear not just in the office but in the real world—and whether they can persist with additional supports.

Finally, it's worth mentioning that the ways in which medication treatments are explained to youth with ADHD can be important for outcome. If the doctor says, essentially, that the medicine should be taken once (or twice, depending on formulation) per day but says nothing else, the child or adult may be led to believe that her own efforts play no role. Yet if the doctor conveys that the medicines will work best only if real effort is put forth—or that the pills may well exert their strongest effects with new and challenging material, or long assignments—and engages your daughter in trying to understand the combination of medication and effort in the process, she should feel far more invested in the whole treatment plan.

Combining Behavioral and Medication Treatments

What if your daughter is participating in an active family/school behavioral program while simultaneously receiving an effective dose of the correct ADHD medication? Wouldn't this combination be optimal? Through medication, the brain should be better attuned for learning thanks to the enhancement of dopamine and norepinephrine functioning in key neural pathways, so that the behavioral intervention can take full effect.

In fact, results from studies of combination treatments (sometimes termed *multimodal interventions*)—compared to effects from either treatment modality alone—are as follows:

- As just noted, symptom reduction gets closer to entering the "normal" range with the combination treatment.

- For outcomes beyond core ADHD symptoms, especially reductions of key associated behaviors (like aggression or depressive mood) along with enhanced academic performance, social skills, and improved parent–child interchanges, the combination is typically superior.

- The psychological and educational effects of behavioral treatments may very well be maximized when the heritable neural expressions of ADHD are offset by effective medication treatment.

But how do the two types of treatments compare when given separately? In head-to-head studies, medications (when optimally adjusted) typically show effects more quickly than do behavioral treatments. In the best-case scenario, stimulants' effects are observable almost immediately. (*Note:* Nonstimulants may take several weeks for full effect; and for youth with the inattentive variety of ADHD, positive effects of any treatment are more subtle and thus harder to discern.) On the other hand, from a behavioral treatment, the rebonding, careful measurement, modeling of a calm approach, deployment of the ABC model, use of rewards and judicious negative consequences, and work with the school may take many weeks for full effect. Furthermore, direct comparisons of medication and behavioral treatment (especially behavioral family therapy) reveal that, for the core symptoms of ADHD (inattention, impulse-control problems, overactivity), medication effects are typically stronger than those from behavioral treatment. Over longer time periods, however, and when considering outcomes and impairments that go beyond symptom reduction per se, behavioral effects on academics, peer relationships, and family interactions may well be just as strong as, if not stronger than, those from medications. Of course, these require real effort from everyone involved.

The bottom line here is that each treatment has advantages—which may be exactly why they work so well together. Interestingly, however, there is some evidence that the timing of treatments can matter. That is, if medications are initiated first, it's harder to find additive effects of behavioral interventions. Yet if the family starts with behavioral treatment—a longer-term process, as just discussed—its effects can be enhanced with effective medication treatment as needed, and perhaps at a lower dose than

> Timing of treatments might matter in terms of the total benefit that your daughter gets from combined medication and behavioral treatment.

what would have been necessary if medication were used alone. Still, the severity of ADHD matters here, such that it may be really important for the most severe cases to have medication treatment instituted sooner rather than later.

Parsing the Decision to Use Medication, with or without Behavioral Treatment

Whether to consider medication for your daughter, with or without behavioral treatment, is a huge question for many if not most families of girls with ADHD. There's so much hype—and so many scare stories about medication as a mind-altering plot against unsuspecting children and families—that it's often difficult to sort out truth from fiction.

Try to think of this issue in the same way you would think about treating high blood pressure. If your primary medical provider puts the blood-pressure cuff on your arm in the office and it's discovered that your reading is 135/85—considered a borderline these days—it might make sense to begin with changes in diet and exercise. But if your initial reading is 280/200, it would undoubtedly be unethical if the doctor didn't start you, right away, on a medication to reduce this blood-pressure reading, given the potential health risks involved. In short, it's all about severity.

So what about ADHD? If the evaluation reveals near- or at-threshold symptoms, with impairment that is potentially manageable, it would probably make sense to start with a course of behavioral family therapy, plus other potential psychosocial treatments. For preschool-age children in particular, the guidelines in the United States and around the world focus on starting with behavioral and psychosocial treatments, as potential effects of medication are weaker than have been demonstrated in older youth, with a higher potential for negative side effects. But if impulsive behavior presents a clear danger, even in a young child, an initial trial of medication may well be in order.

After an evaluation confirming ADHD in your daughter who is beyond the preschool years, what do you say if your doctor recommends starting her on medication right away? Key questions would be as follows: How serious are the potential consequences of her ADHD, for both her and others? Would it make sense to begin with behavioral treatments and then add medication if necessary? What about comorbid behavioral and emotional issues, which should perhaps be addressed first—with different kinds of psychotherapy or medications? In short, there are no simple answers here. Still, ADHD medications have helped countless youth, including girls, with ADHD. And you don't want to wait too long if failure is a regular occurrence.

A few additional points: There are two major "classes" of stimulant medications—the methylphenidate (trade names: Ritalin, Concerta, Focalin, and others) versus amphetamine (trade names: Dexedrine, Adderall, and others) groups. (Again, see the Resources at the back of the book for additional detail.) There is no way to know which class of stimulants, or which dosage, your daughter may respond to optimally, unless you engage in a trial. Such trials should include parent and teacher completion of brief rating scales of ADHD behaviors, tracking of common side effects of the medication, as well as monitoring of behaviors targeted individually to your daughter (which can be added onto a brief ADHD rating scale). All this may take some time and effort, but in the absence of "precision medicine" approaches in the world of ADHD at present, it's the best way forward.

In the end, is it worth it—given the huge debates about the efficacy, and ethics, of ADHD medications—to try? I leave you with this advice: If the behavioral patterns are of significant concern, it might make sense to engage in a trial, with you and the teacher(s) providing ratings, if your provider is equipped to help you manage such a trial. With evidence of real benefit, everyone might win, especially given the data on the optimal efficacy of combining medication with behavioral treatments. If not, at least you can know that a real effort was made to understand that medication was not a viable option. In short, let the evidence speak for itself.

Additional Treatments

As noted earlier, a number of other "treatments" for ADHD are advertised, but few have significant evidence for their effectiveness. The following are the ones that have at least some (if not more) supportive evidence for their use with ADHD.

Organizational Skills Training

The goal here is to help children or teens with ADHD get a handle on organizing their schoolwork/homework and overall lives. How many stories have we all heard about the girl (or boy) with ADHD whose initial week's homework assignment back in August or early September was ultimately found, scrunched and nearly unrecognizable, in her backpack the next spring? Or the bright youth with ADHD who doesn't "get" that one must plan a long-term assignment days or weeks ahead of the final product—with all-nighters rarely producing a good result? Organizational skills training involves kids with ADHD, along with their parents and teachers, in the use of hints, tips, and structure to build on developing executive functions toward the end of greater organization, time estimation and time management, and productivity. Parents and teachers learn to monitor, prompt, and encourage use of binders and other organizational aids, so that youth with ADHD can actually display the intelligence they have and the learning they have done. Organizational skills training is evidence-based, although a major comparative trial showed that effects were similar overall to those from intensive behavioral family therapy.

Aerobic Exercise

It's not much of an exaggeration to say that every animal and human study ever done reveals that exercise improves not only physical functioning but also cognitive performance. But what about ADHD? The headline version here is that a growing set of studies reveals that consistent, at-least-30-minute bouts of aerobic exercise (that is, exercise significantly lifting one's heart rate), several times per week, can help reduce ADHD symptoms and enhance functioning in youth and even adults with ADHD. The effect sizes are small, in comparison with behavioral and medication treatments, but still observable. Thus, it is not mistaken to believe that regular aerobic exercise can and should be a clear part of a holistic treatment program for ADHD.

Neurofeedback

The idea for this treatment modality is that individuals can learn to regulate their mental states and brain functioning through brain-based biofeedback, also called *neurofeedback*. Here the child/teen/adult is engaged in a cognitive task on a computer, while electrodes placed on her scalp link her brain waves to her task performance. When performance and attention are optimal, the feedback provides rewarding sights and sounds. The aim is for girls with ADHD to develop better self-regulation of attention without the intensive coaching and modeling from adults that are an inherent part of behavioral family therapy and school-based therapy.

Initial research revealed that neurofeedback helps individuals with ADHD with respect to attention and self-regulation. However, it could be the case that the computer and scalp-electrode apparatus engenders a large expectancy of positive benefits. In fact, the evidence continues to be mixed: Neurofeedback has been shown to produce medium-sized effects of inattention in several trials—but the latest round of rigorous research shows that it may not outperform a control condition in which the electrodes and feedback are not actually attuned to the individual's actual performance. Despite increasing claims, neurofeedback cannot be recommended as a fully evidence-based intervention for ADHD.

Cognitive and Working Memory Training

During the latter part of the 20th century scientists and clinicians began to posit that, rather than tackling all of the symptoms and impairments related to ADHD at once, perhaps it would be viable to boost some of the underlying executive functioning issues related to ADHD. One of the top contenders was *working memory,* the ability to hold in mind a string of information while also manipulating such information in the service of a goal (think of remembering a phone number before dialing). In fact, working memory is often compromised in individuals with ADHD.

Beginning in Northern Europe and then extending widely, advocates found ways to teach, through memory games and other devices, means of expanding an individual's working memory. With samples composed of youth or adults with ADHD, positive benefits have been found—even extending to alterations in brain networks that appear to underlie efficient working memory. However, the key finding has emerged that despite such gains in the clinic or laboratory, there is very little evidence that these translate into better cognitive or academic or behavioral performance in the real world. In sum, I would not recommend such procedures as any kind of stand-alone treatment for your daughter with ADHD.

Video Games and Apps

We are clearly in an era in which tech-based processes, including an ever-expanding number of apps, are heralded as the solutions for a number of mental-health and neurodevelopmental conditions. Yes, there are some intriguing recent findings: A relatively new video game for ADHD has been shown to increase performance on a highly related measure of computerized vigilance. But at the same time, none of the additional measures of behavioral and cognitive performance at home and school revealed any significant effects. The best term for such games and apps might be *promising,* but they are far from fully validated.

Please see the box on page 148 for additional information on controversial and less substantiated interventions for ADHD.

Treatments for Comorbid Conditions

Remember that ADHD rarely appears as the sole behavioral/emotional condition in need of intervention. A host of linked (called *comorbid*) disorders and conditions can and often do accompany ADHD. In some cases, successful treatment of the underlying ADHD can lessen the burden of such conditions. For example, if one becomes demoralized and even clinically depressed because of the consequences of ADHD in her life, excellent ADHD treatment should lessen such depression. But perhaps the depression and ADHD both emerged during childhood without one clearly preceding the other. Here, and in many other cases, the other condition will require additional treatment strategies that are more closely linked to the specific disorder in question. It would take a book-length account to list each viable intervention for all of the possible disorders frequently linked with ADHD. The best I can do here is highlight just a few examples (see also the Resources at the back of the book).

Depression and Anxiety

CBT for depression, and a different type of psychotherapy called *interpersonal therapy*, are targeted toward youth, teen, or adult depression. As well, SSRI medications, which show little if any benefit for ADHD per se, can be helpful, particularly when combined with the evidence-based psychological treatments for these "internalizing" conditions of depression and anxiety.

Oppositional Defiant Disorder and Conduct Disorder

Oppositional and aggressive behavior patterns tend to respond to the same kinds of behavioral family therapy sessions described earlier in this chapter for ADHD. Furthermore, ADHD medications can help, at least partially, in reducing the impulse-control problems that may contribute to fighting and other signs of aggression. When such "externalizing" behavior reaches more dangerous amounts, higher levels of intervention may be indicated, along with additional medications.

Learning Disorders

Although ADHD treatments can help with the attentional issues that often accompany reading and math disorders in youth, they need to be supplemented with specific academic interventions that give concentrated practice. What's needed is screening/assessment for a learning disorder and then concentrated practice in reading or math or writing, at school and/or via tutoring.

PTSD

As noted above, if a child has been maltreated, trauma-informed psychological therapies are crucial. Yet sometimes trauma does overlap with ADHD—in which case trauma-informed care and ADHD treatment can be combined.

Autism Spectrum Disorders

A decade ago, if a child was diagnosed with an autism spectrum disorder, she couldn't also receive a diagnosis of ADHD. But it's now clearly known that the conditions can overlap. ADHD medications can clearly help with attention- and focus-related problems when comorbidity exists, but they are not effective for the social deficits and problems linked directly to autism. These are optimally treated, as early in life as possible, with intensive in-home behavioral interventions.

Substance Use Disorders

Stimulants can clearly serve as drugs of abuse, so they are often stopped when a teen with ADHD is noted to begin abusing drugs. However, well-monitored ADHD medications (often nonstimulants) can also help with recovery in some cases, when ADHD is also present. Of course, the kinds of rehabilitation and intensive outpatient treatment protocols for substance use and dependence may need to be instituted as well.

Bipolar Disorder and Borderline Personality Disorder

In adolescence (and even in childhood in extreme cases), bipolar disorder can exist, often in tandem with ADHD. If it's clearly present, a mood-stabilizing medication is usually indicated. With such in place, ADHD medications can perhaps be added as well. The family will need psychoeducation related to bipolar disorder, given that its longer-term course can differ from that of ADHD. If borderline personality features emerge, DBT is increasingly evidence-based for such youth, who may also be struggling with many core ADHD symptoms.

More Specialized Behavioral Parent Therapy/ Management Treatments

Parent–child interaction therapy: This is a well-researched form of behavioral parent therapy, designed for preschool- and early-elementary-age children who experience ADHD or oppositional/defiant behavior problems. It is highly structured: In the clinic, parents are observed interacting with their child from behind a one-way mirror as the therapists directly coach them via a small microphone ("bug in the ear") to shape more positive and directive parenting behaviors. It is based directly on teaching authoritative parenting—the combination of warmth/responsiveness and demandingness/limit setting described in Chapter 5—with clear indications of success.

The Child Life and Attention Skills program: This is a comprehensive behavioral family therapy approach designed specifically for children with the inattentive presentation of ADHD. It involves the usual behavioral family therapy principles (yet with more emphasis on skill-building than punishment practices, given that children with primary inattention are not typically aggressive), along with active social skills intervention and parent and teacher involvement. Its main randomized trial revealed clear benefits, over and above behavioral family therapy alone, for home and school issues related to ADHD.

Adolescent adaptations: As described in more detail in Chapter 9, teens often recoil against a straight-up behavioral reward chart, which may seem antiquated or infantilizing for adolescents. Although it would take another book-length account to emphasize fully the kinds of teenage adaptations that are crucial, I can say that behavioral family therapy for adolescents with ADHD feature (1) contracts (rather than reward charts), which emphasize what the teen will do *and* what the parent will do, in terms of expectations and consequences; and (2) the kinds of negotiated give-and-take with respect to independence versus continued family warmth/support needed to propel your daughter into adolescent thriving. The middle-school and high-school years are a time of major surges toward independence in your preteen and teenage daughter, who at the same time must learn to negotiate multiple teachers and multiple subjects each day. As a parent, your own executive functions will be tested to the max as you try to engage the secondary-school setting to support your daughter (see Chapters 7 and 9).

Presence of depression or ADHD in yourself: A lot of important work is being done these days on modifying behavioral parent training for families in which a parent has ADHD or depression. The core idea is that unless these issues are tackled, the parent will not be able to deliver an effective parent management program to her child. Space does not allow full details here, but the pioneering work of Professor Andrea Chronis-Tuscano, at the University of Maryland, provides great guidance in this area (see Further Reading, at the back of the book).

Alternative, Controversial, and Nonsubstantiated Treatments

There are so many "treatments" for ADHD without substantiated evidence that it's hard to know where to begin.

Chiropractic: Adjusting the spine might help with back pain or related issues, but there's no substantial evidence at all that it makes even a dent with respect to ADHD symptoms and impairments.

Diet: Isn't ADHD curable via alterations in the foods we eat? Of course, many of us could eat healthier diets than we typically do. But the former claims of the Feingold diet, and other such regimens, have simply not withstood careful clinical trials. Still, evidence exists that dyes and additives, especially for children with ADHD, may exacerbate some symptoms. The bottom line: A healthy diet may well be part of a holistic treatment regimen for ADHD, but changing diet alone is not an evidence-based intervention for individuals with this diagnosis.

Supplements: So many nonmonitored or unregulated supplements are touted as treatments for ADHD, but few have even a shred of evidence. Yet omega-3 oils, often found in certain fish or via supplements, may well help with underlying neural foundations. Recent trials suggest a small, slow-to-emerge, but detectable effect.

SEVEN

Educating Your Daughter with ADHD

Ensuring their daughter's education is a major concern for most parents of girls with ADHD. As earlier chapters have explained, ADHD can interfere with academic performance in a variety of ways, and the social challenges raised by ADHD can create problems in the classroom and in girls' relationships with classmates. This chapter is intended to provide the information and advice you need to ease your daughter's path through school, from kindergarten through high school. Note, though, that this chapter focuses mainly on the academic aspects of schooling. Chapter 8 deals with young girls with ADHD, including their social worlds and social interactions—at home, in the neighborhood, and at school; Chapter 9 does the same for adolescent girls with ADHD.

So, in the following pages, I address two key questions:

1. What kind of school would be best, taking into account both your daughter's symptoms and impairments and accommodations that different types of schools may offer?

2. Which kinds of behavioral and academic programs, coordinated between school and home, will help your daughter with ADHD the most?

First, please understand that these two topics are naturally interrelated. You can't judge a school without knowing what types of programs it offers, and you can't expect any school to do everything to ensure a good education for your daughter. In short, you'll need to play an active role.

Second, there is no single, all-encompassing answer to the question of what type of school will be best for your daughter. You now know that there are huge individual differences among females diagnosed with this condition, so what works for your daughter with ADHD will not necessarily be the school that your neighbor's daughter thrives in, or the one that's great for your cousin's daughter, even though they both have ADHD as well. Indeed, a whole lot depends on the relationship you develop with the teachers and administrators of whatever school your child attends, especially the ways in which home and school behavioral programs are coordinated.

Third, let me tip you off to one of my underlying beliefs: Based on my clinical and research experience, I am convinced that a large number of girls with ADHD can thrive in regular classrooms in public-school settings. *Yet they can do so only if effective home–school communication, collaboration, and reward programs are established.* For girls with more severe ADHD symptoms, and/or comorbid disorders requiring additional interventions, it may be necessary to add other supports and accommodations, including some "pull-out" resource classrooms, all the way to out-of-public-school placements. Again, a whole lot depends on your daughter's strengths and weaknesses, your tenacity in procuring accommodations (and even more, evidence-based treatments), the willingness of teachers and other school personnel to get on board, and your sense of the best environments for your daughter as she matures. Also keep in mind the somewhat unavoidable trade-offs: Specialized schools/programs can provide more individualized attention but may also restrict your daughter's chances for peer interactions (for example, think of homeschooling that doesn't involve plentiful outings with other kids). A regular classroom setting offers daily interaction with many agemates—but, as I just noted, it can be productive only if needed supports are arranged.

Fourth, I can't overstate the importance of active collaboration between you and your daughter's school. The behavioral programs, promotion of better executive functions and academic output, and teacher-specific encouragement for your daughter that a school should offer all rely on your own efforts to make these provisions work. These are essential parts of a comprehensive plan to help your

> *Even the best comprehensive program available won't help your daughter thrive in school without your collaboration and communication.*

daughter thrive, regardless of the particular type of school she attends. Indeed, as emphasized in Chapter 6, a viable family intervention program for girls with ADHD must include regular, consistent contact with teachers and schools. The sheer need for consistency in the life of your daughter mandates that comprehensive intervention programs include explicit communication and coordination with her school. After all, academic underperformance is arguably *the* core area of impairment for girls with ADHD. In fact, research documents that girls with ADHD underperform in academics far more than do typically developing girls—and even more so than boys with ADHD do, particularly in math.

Finally, you'll notice in the pages that follow that I highlight certain essentials, no matter what school your daughter attends: (1) regular rewards for your daughter's sticking with the program prescribed (the daily report card sent home by teachers, discussed below, is an important tool here) and (2) assistance with her development of organizational skills and executive functions. Growth in organizational abilities and executive functions may well be the core of your daughter's burgeoning academic and self-regulatory success. Although social problems in the school setting are also crucial for girls with ADHD, I save discussion of peer-related difficulties for Chapters 8 and 9.

Which Kinds of Schools?

Before I discuss various schooling options, it's necessary to start off with information about your daughter's potential access to accommodations. As will become clear, not all types of schools can or will provide accommodations. The more you know at the outset, the better prepared you should be.

Accommodations

The legal rights of children experiencing disabilities—along with their families—have expanded enormously over the past half century in the United States. Before the 1970s, huge numbers of children and adolescents with all sorts of disabilities—sensory, physical, neurodevelopmental—did not have any mandated access to public schooling. To promote such access, public-school districts have been and are now required to provide appropriate accommodations at no cost to families. Short of making this chapter a legal document, here's a summation.

The Individuals with Disabilities Education Act (IDEA)

Under IDEA, all students with documented disabilities are entitled to a free public education, via provision of special-education-related accommodations. Think, for example, of a hearing-impaired child, who may perform optimally, depending on the severity of the impairment, with low background noise, assistive listening devices, interpreters, and/or remote captioning. Youth with visual impairments could require notes and handouts in Braille, or tactiled (sometimes called "haptic") printed materials. Parallels for a girl with ADHD might include classroom supports/accommodations such as a better student–teacher ratio, extra time on certain assignments or tests (though this is not as essential as some believe, as noted later), being seated directly in front of the teacher, directions that are presented both visually and orally, special binders for organizational purposes, more frequent rewards, and a host of additional ones. The second half of this chapter discusses these in more detail.

Under this landmark federal law, all students with disabilities age 3–21 years are entitled to a Free Appropriate Public Education (with the acronym of FAPE). *Free* really does mean "free"—there is no tuition for a FAPE. The original version of this statute appeared in 1975 as the Education for All Handicapped Children Act. During its subsequent reauthorizations, with the name change to IDEA, the diagnosis of ADHD became listed formally as one of the specific disabilities that could qualify a student for special educational services (that is, as one of several "Other Health Impaired" conditions).

Overall, there must be clear documentation that the child or adolescent (1) has a disability (in accordance with specific lists in the statute, such as ADHD)—but one that (2) affects their educational attainment or ability to benefit from the general curriculum in regular-education classrooms. In other words, a disability alone is a necessary but not a sufficient condition: Whatever the disability, it must also require the need for specialized instruction.

To document the disability, school personnel need to administer evaluations and tests. Sometimes, outside evaluators are called upon.

The family and district then work together to form an individualized education program (IEP), which lays out the target goals and related accommodations to meet those goals. The IEP includes the kind of classroom and school settings required to enact specific learning objectives. For instance, an IEP for a girl with ADHD may specify certain lengths of time she should be able to remain seated for certain activities—or the kinds of academic progress in specific target areas that should be expected over the next school year. There are clear guidelines as to who must be on an IEP team: a parent/caregiver, at least one of the child's general education teachers, at least one special education teacher, a school psychologist or other specialist who can interpret evaluation findings, and a district representative with authority over special education services. The IEP is a legally binding document, with the inclusion of measurable outcomes to denote progress, plus periodic review.

An underlying principle is that, for eligible students, placements should be in the "least restrictive environment" that can provide a free education in sync with the student's needs. That is, needed supports in a regular classroom setting receive priority over a fully separate classroom, or a separate school, unless adequate supports and accommodations are simply not available in the less restrictive alternative.

IDEA is a huge step forward. Indeed, millions of children formerly without access to a public education can now receive one. Over the years IDEA has expanded to cover the following:

- Financial grants to preschools to assist with special education for 3- to 5-year-olds
- Identifying infants and toddlers with disabilities
- Assisted technology services for many children with physical, sensory, or neurodevelopmental conditions
- Coverage through a student's 22nd birthday (as long as the individual is still in public secondary schooling)

For an overview, see the website *www.seewritehear.com/learn/individuals-with-disabilities-education-act-idea*.

Yet things do not always go smoothly in the IEP process. Although IDEA guarantees a FAPE, the statute is what's called an *underfunded mandate*. In other words, the federal government does not cover all costs associated with a FAPE. In fact, although the initial intention was for approximately 40% of such costs to be federally covered, this goal was never obtainable, and the actual reimbursement is now under 20%. Thus, local districts and their accompanying states must pick up the tab, at a point in history when public education is receiving far less rather than more state support. As a result, legal battles for the needed types of accommodations and placements, especially those outside of

Although IDEA mandates "free" education, the reality is that the mandate is underfunded—not just federally but by the states and local school districts left with filling the gap. So be prepared for negotiations and even legal battles to get the accommodations your daughter needs.

regular classrooms, can become protracted and heated. Provisions of IDEA call for mediation as needed, but attorneys can and do get involved in formal lawsuits. In short, parents of girls with ADHD must sometimes engage in extended negotiations and legal battles to obtain desired accommodations and programs.

Section 504

Another avenue for accommodations is Section 504 of the federal Rehabilitation Act of 1973, administered by the federal Office for Civil Rights. This statute prohibits discrimination with respect to disability, in any programs or activities that receive any amount of funding from the U.S. Department of Education—including just about all public schools. It is an antidiscrimination law, meaning that (unlike IDEA) it does not target special education per se. Even more, it does not provide funds for services. Still, families may sue a district for failing to provide accommodations for a student with a disability, so that at least some accountability is present.

An evaluation must document a physical or mental impairment—including emotional, mental, or learning disorders, which could include ADHD—that substantially limits a major life activity, such as concentrating, thinking, and/or reading. Teams enacting the resultant 504 plans are smaller and less stringently mandated than are IEP teams. Moreover, 504 plans lack the same IEP requirements for measured growth during the follow-up period. In general, such plans focus on changes in the learning environment to prevent discrimination, whereas IEPs can mandate actual special education procedures to meet the specific learning needs of a particular child. Because Section 504 has a broader definition of a disability than IDEA, youth who fail to qualify for an IEP may still qualify for a 504 plan. For a convenient table of key differences between IEPs and 504 plans, see *https://understood.org/articles/en/the-difference-between-ieps-and-504-plans*.

Keep this legal information in mind as you read the following descriptions of four major schooling options for all youth, including those with ADHD: public schools, charter schools, private schools, and homeschooling. I include information about which kinds of accommodations may be available in each.

Public Schools

In the United States, as well as many other countries, the default is that your daughter will attend public school. By definition, such schools receive support from taxpayer dollars in particular school districts as well as from overall state funds, with a small amount of federal support as well. Each public-school district must serve all youth within that district and strictly follow curriculum guidelines from its respective state board of education. However, given the different property tax rates in wealthy versus poorer communities, affluent areas have greater funding levels for public schools, with direct implications for both regular education and special education.

Indeed, classroom size in many public schools has grown increasingly large, especially in less affluent districts and as state support levels dwindle. Many parents must therefore decide whether a smaller class would be optimal for their daughter with ADHD via other options. Yet, as discussed below, private schools can be extremely expensive, and they are not mandated to provide accommodations.

By definition, any public-school student with a documented disability may be eligible for an IEP under IDEA, as well as a 504 plan. (However, if a student gets an IEP, it may not be worth fighting for a 504 plan as well, as the IEP is usually more stringent and comprehensive.) Battle lines can be drawn as district administrators strain to make their budgets operative for both regular and special education. There are real fiscal limits on the number, and types, of accommodations for students with ADHD, which remains a stigmatized, underappreciated, and undervalued disability.

Charter Schools

Charter schools are a real hybrid. Although publicly funded, they are operated as independent entities—or at least semi-independent, depending on the state and district—under a specific charter for a particular educational purpose. So, they are not private; instead, they operate with public funds for a specific purpose. Most are nonprofit, but a minority operate on a for-profit basis. There is no tuition.

Such schools are typically smaller than regular public schools, with more flexibility, because they are not subject to the strict curricula of state boards of education or local districts. Many, in fact, are specialized, with a particular focus (for example, arts); thus, they don't offer the standard options (with many electives) of "true" public schools, especially at the high-school level. Some charter schools may not be willing to accept children with disabilities or special needs, which would increase their operating costs. Yet all must adhere to their specific charter; otherwise, they can lose their public funding. For a guide, see *https://edweek.org/policy-politics/what-are-charter-schools/2018/08*.

What about accommodations? Because of their receipt of public funding, charter schools must respect IEPs and deliver required accommodations. In most situations, they must also operate in accordance with 504 plans.

Private Schools

Private schools are, by definition, privately owned and operated. (Included here are parochial schools.) Admission is selective, and tuition can be steep. Most private schools aim to promote academic achievement in a setting with a more favorable student–teacher ratio than available in typical public-school classrooms. Accordingly, many private schools may be unwilling to accept students with known disabilities, who could, in their view, require services not available to the other students in the classroom or school.

> *Private schools specializing in ADHD can offer low teacher–student ratios and other desirable accommodations, but because they generally are not mandated to do so by IDEA and not publicly funded, the positives often come at a high financial cost to families.*

Overall, there is no federal mandate for private schools to offer the kinds of accommodations or supports required of publicly funded or charter schools. It's worth checking into specific options, however, because there are occasional exceptions:

- Some private schools may in fact receive some amount of public funding and thus be mandated for accommodations.
- Since 2004, reauthorizations of IDEA have tried to encourage the

provision of at least some special services for disabled youth in private schools.

- Although it's extremely rare given the costs, an IEP created for a girl with severe ADHD (or other conditions) may include funding for private schooling.

On the other hand, some private schools, whether day schools or residential, specialize in disorders like ADHD, with favorable student–teacher ratios. The costs, as a result, are often extremely high.

Homeschooling

Homeschooling is an option for a number of families of children with or without disabilities. The child does not attend a traditional school but learns at home, under the guidance of a parent/teacher, sometimes with several children from other families. Different states have widely varied statutes governing homeschooling, with some requiring credentials for teachers but others having few if any such requirements. Many homeschooled children, and the parents who teach them, receive guidance from state and national standards, which cover planning of lessons, assigning of homework, and grading. After a surge in numbers of homeschooled youth during the late 1990s and early 2000s, the numbers have leveled off at around 2% of school-age children and adolescents.

Some advocates promote this method for girls with ADHD, as it clearly provides for more individualized attention, prevents the rules and strictures of most schools (for example, needing to sit down for long periods of time), may prevent bullying and other negative peer interactions, and could help the girl discover natural abilities and talents. Disadvantages include the lack of built-in agemates in public or private schooling and, of course, the huge time and energy investments involved for the parents who perform the teaching. Note that many homeschooled children actually do participate in group activities (for example, at museums or on sports teams), so it's mistaken to believe that homeschooling is always a completely isolated activity. Of course, without controlled research—randomly assigning some children to public schools and others to homeschooling, which is pretty much impossible to do—whether longer-term gains in academics and social skills accrue from homeschooling is unknown. For a guide, see *https://additudemag.com/unschooling-homeschooling-adhd-learning-strategies*.

Of course, during the COVID-19 pandemic, homeschooling took on a whole new meaning, as most children in the United States were "schooled" at home, often via remote learning, with increased demands on parents to monitor schoolwork and homework. Girls and boys with ADHD clearly experienced challenges in such a virtual environment. Undoubtedly, the experience also gave many parents a taste for what teachers instructing students with ADHD encounter on a day-by-day basis.

It should go without saying, but I'll say it nonetheless: Homeschooling is not a publicly supported form of education. Not surprisingly, then, no mandated accommodations are available.

Please see the box on page 159 about recent research on accommodations for ADHD—which may not always yield the kinds of benefits that were intended.

What's Best?

As noted at the start of the chapter, there's no single or simple answer here. In fact, parents of youth with ADHD are often perplexed as to the best option. *ADDitude* magazine conducted and then reported on a survey of nearly 1,000 parents of special-needs children, with around half of the families raising a child with ADHD. Incredibly, fully 100% of the caregivers of kids with ADHD said they had considered changing schools for their child—and 63% had already made a school switch at the time of the survey! Key reasons cited were related to the relative inflexibility of public-school curricula, the lack of ability of school personnel to manage behavior challenges (whether at public or private schools), or the child's anxiety over schooling. Clearly, decisions in this domain are far from easy.

For a summary, see *https://additudemag.com/best-schools-for-adhd-children-change-survey*.

To help frame the debate, let's briefly review the core academic needs of girls with ADHD:

- Support and positive encouragement
- Structure (in terms of time, assignments, and expectations)
- Small steps toward success

ADHD Accommodations:
Be Careful What You Wish For?

Do most accommodations for ADHD, as enacted in IEPs or 504 plans, really "work"? That is, do they lead to skill gains for students diagnosed with ADHD? A recent review article (see Lovett and Nelson in the Further Reading section for this chapter) provides some real food for thought.

First, accommodations for students with ADHD are widespread, both for instruction and for testing. Extended time on tests is extremely common. Also frequent are reduced expectations for homework completion.

Second, and crucially, there is extremely little research that supports the benefits of accommodations for grades, test scores, and the like regarding children with ADHD. In existing studies, some accommodations (for example, teaching or testing in small groups; extended time) are not supported at all or barely supported. The exception here, for early-primary-grade students with ADHD, is that test instructions that are read out loud by the teacher may provide benefit.

Third, many of the common accommodations for youth with ADHD do not appear to be at all specific to such youth but would probably assist any student. So, there would be no special gains for students with ADHD.

Fourth, and also important to note, accommodations may in many cases take the place of actual behavioral interventions (for example, for organizational skills and time management, or specific academic remediation, or even medication). This is not a good state of affairs! In other words, if lowered expectations are the main "message" of accommodations, rather than the use of programs or interventions that can build skills, they could be self-defeating.

Finally, many students with ADHD, as well as educational professionals, have voiced skepticism about the actual value of many accommodations (for example, extended testing time), if they lead to lowered expectations or if teachers believe that such accommodations will be difficult to implement.

Much more research needs to be done on specific accommodations—and specific classroom teaching procedures—with respect to benefits for girls and boys with ADHD. But this research provides a warning that accommodations for many youth with ADHD may not be providing expected benefits, or actually could be counterproductive, if they take the place of needed behavioral programs and academic remediation. Perhaps accommodations should be more time-limited (that is, not "permanent" over many years), so that evidence-based treatments can be allowed to work.

My goal in providing this information is not to discourage your seeking of needed accommodations but to make sure that strong educational and behavioral programs—as discussed in the second half of this chapter—are the primary focus.

- Extrinsic motivation programs, including positive contingencies (rewards), which should be individualized to the greatest extent possible
- Teaching of organizational and executive skills
- Prompting of the kinds of executive functions that could help her with self-regulation

A key question is whether these kinds of needs can be attained within the large class sizes characteristic of many public schools. One answer here is whether the family can secure accommodations and, even more, needed treatments. Additionally, I pose several questions to you:

- What are your values with respect to public versus private education?
- What can you afford?
- How willing (and able) are you to work with teachers on school-based classroom management programs, coordinated with your home behavioral program?
- How hard are you willing to fight for formal accommodations and/or treatment strategies, and at what cost if agreement is not reached?

An important perspective here pertains to optimal classroom styles for youth with ADHD. A truly interesting perspective, based on real evidence, is that the best blend combines the elements of *informal* and *structured*. Although this conjunction may seem counterintuitive, let me explain.

A formal classroom is one in which the student is expected to sit all day for a lecture-style approach from the teacher. Such formality doesn't play to the strengths of a girl with ADHD and may actually clash with such strengths. In other words, building in frequent breaks, allowing her to stand for certain assignments, and providing opportunities for different kinds of learning (individual, classroom-as-a whole, peer tutoring, small group) appear to be optimal for many girls (and boys) with ADHD. Hence, the *informal* approach may be optimal.

At the same time, however, clear expectations and limits should be present. High levels of *structure* and guidance, including clear expectations, are ideal. Indeed, a classroom setting that lacks cues, schedules, highly organized materials, "chunked" assignments, and frequent rewards may be nearly impossible for kids with ADHD to negotiate with success. In fact, a truly unstructured approach (what used to be called "open classrooms") may mask a girl's ADHD in the sense that no one in the classroom is sitting—all are pursuing individual choices. Yet her learning of academics and self-regulation is likely to be seriously compromised. Structure, within a setting that allows for individual differences in learning styles, may well be the ideal.

If you're seeing parallels here with authoritative parenting—the blend of warmth and support with structure and control—you are on the right track. For helpful information in this regard, see *www.familyeducation.com/school/ classroom-modifications/best-classrooms-children-adhd.*

And, for an interesting "grading" of the relative benefits of public versus private versus homeschooling options for youth with ADHD, see *https://study. com/blog/considerations-for-picking-the-best-school-for-your-adhd-child.html.*

Finally, for one family's views on the relative benefits of public versus private school for their daughter with ADHD, please see the box on page 162.

At this point we're ready to discuss coordinating family behavioral programs with school-based management. The core question is as follows: Given what you've just read, what must you do to extend the principles and steps of behavioral family therapy, discussed in Chapter 6, to ensure coordinated efforts and parallel programs facilitated by your daughter's teachers at whatever school she attends?

Integration of Home and School Behavioral Programs

Let's get right to it: Girls with ADHD require as much consistency as possible across expectations, tasks, and settings. In other words, despite your strong efforts to reward her successive steps toward better behavior at home, as well as performance in homework, what will happen if your daughter receives quite a different set of antecedents and consequences at school? You probably know the answer already: Her performance will suffer, and any chances for home–school coordination will be lost.

The best behavioral family therapy programs for ADHD include explicit instruction in how to connect with teachers, initiate parent–teacher meetings

Public versus Private School Decision: Another Perspective

Parents of students with ADHD, whether girls or boys, strongly consider changing school placements—or actually do so. Such decisions place a huge weight on families, who must debate the pros and cons of which type of school is best, without sound knowledge to guide them. These decisions also strain the child, for sure, as switching schools can disrupt peer relationships and the environment created by the former teacher.

Of course, economic factors are a huge concern here, given the extremely high costs of many private school options as an alternative to public schools. *ADDitude* magazine provided a personal account of one family's struggles around the issue of private versus public school for their daughter with ADHD–Inattentive. The tagline for this account is as follows:

Academically, private school was the best choice for our daughter. She is a different learner who benefits enormously from small classes and individual attention. Socially, however, the departure from public school has been quite another story.

In short, while trying to configure the best learning environment for their daughter, the family witnessed, in the transfer to a private school, real erosion of peer supports along with the sheer time involved in driving her to and from the new school. They were sure that the particular private school they'd located was optimal for her academically—but was it worth the long commute, their daughter's lack of time with peers in the neighborhood, her exhaustion from studies, and family stress related to all of the above? Clearly, any decision involves trade-offs.

For the full report, please see *https://additudemag.com/private-school-vs-public-school.*

(which may also be attended by your behavioral therapist, at least initially), coordinate home and school goals, and work on making rewards for your daughter's behavior and her academic performance as consistent as possible across your home and her classroom.

In public and charter school settings, if your daughter has an IEP or a 504 plan, it's far easier to get your daughter's teacher (or teachers, plural, in most middle and high schools) to "enlist," as the accommodations in her plan are mandatory. But it's important to keep in mind that, whether or not she has an IEP/504 plan in place, teachers have multiple students throughout a day, and many need sensitive education as to your daughter's needs as well as those of other kids with ADHD. Not to mention other needs of other children in the class. Respect for the teacher's multiple roles can go a long way. In fact, when teachers gain skills in behavioral classroom management, all students in the class may benefit. Still, as noted earlier in this chapter, conflicts can occur, and some schools/teachers may believe that you're simply coddling a girl cavalierly who has been diagnosed with something called ADHD—but who is not really trying. An approach that appeals to the teacher's empathy, along with the teacher's desire to follow federal law if formal accommodations are granted, may well be optimal.

General Plans

As your home behavioral program is developing (see Chapter 6)—including behaviorally specific goals, the ABC model, and a reward system—it's time to set up meetings with your daughter's teacher. In these conferences, the initial aims are to inform the teacher of your knowledge of your daughter and to help instill the sense that she needs a more regular and structured set of guidelines and expectations each school day. If you have one, you should also review the specific accommodations listed in the IEP or 504 plan for her.

Some basic classroom adaptations are as follows, by rough categories. They are worded to speak directly to teachers; you can pass them on in your communications with your daughter's teacher.

Seating

Make sure that the girl with ADHD is seated front and center, in the teacher's direct line of sight. This simple step can minimize distractions and allow the teacher to prompt and cue such a girl more regularly. As an aside, I remember some years back, when the rage in northern California elementary schools was to have circular or oval tables of 5 or 6 children each, spread throughout the classroom. An interesting idea, for sure, in terms of promoting group work—except that a number of children with ADHD may have been facing away from the teacher for an entire semester!

Another related idea is to pair, at a table, a girl with ADHD with a peer displaying greater self-regulation, as a model.

Instructions

Make them basic, clear, and concise. Provide them across multiple modalities—that is, on the board, orally, and online.

Assignments

Consider "chunking" them into smaller units and consider allowing extra time for completion. (Although the box above cautions that if the only adjustments or accommodations for your daughter are for extended time, the benefits may be limited.) Be flexible with respect to homework demands. When appropriate, use timers to assist the student with remembering to complete work.

Cueing

Let students know what's expected. Have a special signal for the teacher to prompt to pay particular attention or stay on task. A gentle tap on shoulder could assist with cues.

Praise and Rewards

Use plentifully! Reward small steps. Provide immediate feedback when possible. Be encouraging. Provide reassurance.

Negative Consequences

Ignore minor inappropriate behavior. Avoid lecturing and/or undue criticism. Provide corrective feedback privately rather than in front of the whole class.

Organization

Use assignment notebooks and electronic calendars. Color-code materials by subject matter. Provide assistance with note-taking (for older students), as appropriate. For long-term assignments, make sure that the student can break the tasks down into component parts.

Flexibility

Allow standing at times, rather than constant sitting. Provide breaks as needed. Understand that the girl with ADHD may not conform in lock-step the way that most of her peers can.

Positive Peer Regard

Provide leadership and/or prominent roles so that classmates can see the girl in a more positive light.

This is a brief sampling. For a list of 72 common classroom adaptations and informal accommodations, see *https://prntexas.org/wp-content/uploads/2017/11/72-Accommodations-That-Can-Help-Students-with-ADHD-TA.pdf.*

Daily Report Card

There's a crucial, evidence-based element for any coordinated home–school program, called a *daily report card (DRC)*. The fundamental idea is to extend your daughter's home reward program into the classroom. That is, you and the teacher (or teacher's aide, or other key adults in contact with your daughter at school) need to "conference" to come up with initial classroom goals, termed *target behaviors*. They should be in the general areas of (1) academic performance, (2) behavior management, and (3) peer relationships. Just as in your home reward program, these targets need to be worded as specifically as possible—and broken down into small, achievable steps, especially at the beginning. No one may agree on what "being more cooperative" really entails. Instead, specific acts of sharing, or amounts of time listening to others' conversations, are far more specific and measurable.

> The daily report card is one of the most powerful tools you have—as long as it's used collaboratively by you and your daughter's teachers.

I can't emphasize enough the importance of starting *small* and with *attainable* goals. That is, your daughter should begin with one or two academic goals, one or two behavioral goals, and perhaps initially a single peer-related goal, with each targeted for a level of at least a 75% chance of success. In other words, don't make them so difficult that she will frequently fail. Crucially, it's essential to word each goal in such a way that the teacher can rate her via a simple *yes* or *no*. For example, during reading circle, an initial goal might be for her to participate for 10 minutes (up from the 6 or 7 minutes she typically lasts). Alternatively, she participates with three or fewer teacher reminders to stay on task. Then, at the end of that circle time, the teacher can easily indicate whether she did or did not meet her goal that day, via a simple circling of the *yes* or *no* column on the DRC.

The transition to home is then crucial: At the end of the school day, your daughter brings the DRC back to you—and you tally her *yes* responses on her home reward chart. (Of course, e-mail or texting can now substitute for the tried-and-true paper DRC sheets or index cards.) The more *yes*es, the more points she earns, tradable for either immediate (small), intermediate, or longer-term (larger) rewards.

What does all this do? First, it ensures that you and your daughter's teacher (plus other school personnel) are aligned—and allied—with respect to her performance in the academic setting. Second, it assures consistency, in that the rewards your daughter receives at home are now contingent on her performance both at home *and* at school. Third, it helps continued monitoring of her progress throughout the day. That is, it serves as a vehicle for continued communication and collaboration.

Once your daughter is in middle school or high school, things get more complex, given the range of subjects and teachers she now has. At a technical level, it's not difficult to configure a DRC for each class—or a more generalized DRC, with each subject/teacher in a different column. Yet it certainly takes more coordination on your (and your daughter's) part to make it work. Note that Chapter 9 provides specific information on working with adolescent girls with ADHD in a variety of settings.

For additional issues and details about DRCs, please see the box on pages 167–168. The crucial point is that DRCs have been shown to be truly effective, if willingness, coordination, and follow-through are all in place.

Teaching and Training for Development of Classroom Skills and Executive Functions

As described early in this book, executive functions are those essential higher-order cognitive skills that relate to "masterminding" one's approach to new activities and new tasks, problems to be solved, and negotiating the distractions

A Few Tips for Success with Your Daughter's DRC

A host of research studies have shown the value of DRCs in promoting better behavior and better academic performance at school and at home. Here are a few additional suggestions for making the most of this tool.

1. If you're worried that your daughter's disorganization will make it tough for the DRC to reach your home each afternoon, you might start with a clear target goal: the DRC gets into the backpack and makes it home in one piece! As well, the cyber world can assist, with DRC *yes* and *no* responses transmitted via text or e-mail attachment, as noted in this chapter.

2. Once the initial DRC is established and beginning to reveal progress, consider adding or substituting additional target behaviors. But remember, the aim is not to have an encyclopedia-length list of such behaviors. Keep it simple. Once a given target is mastered, it's time to sub in another.

3. Over time, aim at a wider range of targets, as ADHD probably causes your daughter problems in most domains of life. Examples include:

- Outdoor/playground (for example, "follows rules and refrains from fighting after lunch while on yard")
- Behavior during a time-out (for example, "serves time-out with no yelling or arguing")
- Taking care of belongings (for example, "places jacket/backpack in appropriate spaces with X or fewer reminders")
- Additional aspects of peer interactions (for example, "does not bother classmates during work periods"; "ignores being provoked by classmate")

4. For a creative extension of a DRC—with a willing and motivated teacher—consider the following. Not only does your daughter bring her DRC home each day to be added to your household reward program, but you add "rows" on the bottom of the DRC for key target behaviors *at home*, for which you add a *yes* or *no* response in the evening. She then takes the DRC back to school each day, and the teacher counts the *yes* responses, adding them to your daughter's classroom reward chart. Such a "reverse DRC" is not always attainable—the teacher may not have the bandwidth for an individualized reward chart for each child with ADHD in the class—but think of the advantages of doing so. That is, the consistency of expectations for performance now goes both ways, school-to-home and home-to-school.

5. For extremely helpful guides to DRCs, see *https://addituemag.com/ daily-report-card-to-improve-adhd-classroom-behavior* and *https://ccf.fiu. edu/research/_assets/how_to_establish_a_school_drc.pdf*.

Importantly, the latter document includes a list, at the end, of issues to consider for troubleshooting a home–school DRC program that isn't gaining needed traction. This list includes reminders about the attainability of initial target behaviors, the provision of visual prompts throughout the day to remind your daughter of her objectives, making sure that there is a reward "menu" at home, and many more.

and inevitable errors that occur. By definition, they are broader and more all-encompassing than specific cognitive knowledge of, say, a given academic subject or a given behavioral goal. They help each and all of us approach the vagaries and complexities of life. Included are planning, inhibition of task-irrelevant thoughts or impulses, working memory (holding on to and manipulating several bits of information at once), error detection and correction, staying persistent in the face of distractions, changing "set" when task demands change, and the like. As ADHD expert Russell Barkley states, core deficits in such functions predict impairments in five core areas linked to self-control:

1. Self-motivation

2. Self-restraint

3. Self-management in relation to time

4. Self-organization

5. Self-regulation of emotions

Although not every girl or boy with ADHD has executive function problems, the majority do, often at moderate to severe levels. No wonder that self-regulation is a core theme for girls with ADHD. Steps at school to minimize the impact of executive function problems and remediate them are extremely important. As noted in Chapter 6, until your daughter is in mid- to late adolescence and then heading toward adulthood, one-on-one cognitive-behavioral strategies are not terribly effective in this regard. Instead, altering contingencies in the classroom environment plays a key role in both sculpting the development of higher levels of executive functioning and aiding in your daughter's ability to stay engaged throughout a school day. Some examples follow.

- Provide external cues relevant to the task at hand, while removing distracting cues. Getting the student's eye contact, and pointing/showing beyond a verbal explanation, can really help here.

- Make "time" cues visible as well, via timelines and calendars, drawing in your daughter to focus on the immediate goals, not the distant ones. Along these lines, provide guidance with projects involving extended time (for example, a week- or month-long task). Try to keep instructions and rewards as focused on today's task as possible.

- As emphasized throughout the book, provide extrinsic rewards, because of the omnipresent deficit in generation of intrinsic motivation for girls with ADHD.

- Relatedly, be aware of the kinds of tasks that are particularly challenging for girls (and boys) with ADHD, because they do not generate large amounts of intrinsic engagement. In particular, such tasks include those that (1) are rote, (2) require substantial independence, (3) are involved with waiting and delays, (4) mandate sitting for long periods of time, and (5) are truly challenging and multifaceted. Such tasks are the kinds for which the student with ADHD will need the most assistance.

- Add physical modalities to learning—for example, when your daughter is initially learning arithmetic skills, allow the use of objects to be counted rather than insisting on strictly mental work. Or, to generate ideas for a project, have her write the ideas on index cards or a computer file before having her attempt to organize them.

- As for transitions, watch out! By the end of a school period, girls with ADHD may have finally become in tune with their current class unit or activity. But when the bell sounds or the teacher announces a switch, things can go haywire in a hurry. Helping to plan explicitly for transitions is another way of scaffolding better executive functioning. In a proactive way, the teacher explicitly asks the girl to stop her current activity, then announces a couple of key rules and expectations for the new activity (and, importantly, has her repeat those rules back), explains the reward/negative consequence contingencies for this activity, and finally instructs her to begin.

- Try to alternate high-interest/high-appeal lessons and activities with more rote/routine ones. Asking for a ton of low-appeal work all morning is bound to "try" the attention and motivation of any student but particularly one with ADHD.

- Assign smaller units or "bursts" of schoolwork expectations with relatively frequent breaks. The goal is not to lower such expectations altogether, but rather to align expectations with the impairments related to ADHD.

Some Educational Realities for Girls with ADHD

Most of the information above could pertain equally well to girls and boys with ADHD. But there are some differences regarding girls that you should be aware of so that you can get the best education possible for your daughter. Many girls with ADHD have ways of hiding/minimizing their symptoms while at the same time internalizing the toll that the symptoms incur. And, as emphasized throughout the book, girls are more likely than boys are to display the inattentive presentation of ADHD, with subtler and easier-to-miss (or misinterpret) symptoms.

Adaptations and Accommodations: Potentially Harder to Obtain?

We're now well into the third decade of the 21st century. Yet despite considerable progress, there's *still* a bias in the field that girls don't show ADHD nearly as much as boys. When symptoms are present, there's usually another explanation for them (for example, anxiety, depression, conduct problems, misapplied gender roles, a lack of trying, and many more). As a result, it may take far more documentation to, and convincing of, school personnel that your daughter truly has ADHD.

Under IDEA, the school district leads the way in performing the assessment and evaluation of whether your daughter qualifies for an IEP, along with the special educational accommodations and services it provides. Even though you may have worked hard to engage assessors in evaluating and diagnosing your daughter, the district may decide that its own assessment is more pertinent. In fact, I know of school districts in California that have their own explicit guidelines on what constitutes ADHD. In some of these districts, the guidelines essentially ignore the inattentive symptoms and focus nearly exclusively on impulsive and disruptive behaviors. Little wonder that girls' accommodations are limited and their learning needs are ignored. Be prepared to be assertive in defending the validity of the inattentive form of ADHD as a truly impairing condition. Emphasize the reality of your daughter's symptoms—even though they may be "masked," at least in part, by her expected gender role or her high levels of compensatory strategies (such as super-high levels of trying, which come at great cost to her sense of self-worth and even her health).

Progress: Potentially Harder to Measure?

If you're a boy with the combined form of ADHD, it's easy for almost anyone to notice your prowess at spitball throwing, your loud assertions that your class-room and home problems are everyone else's fault, and your overtly physical approach to life. If you make progress, nearly everyone will quickly notice. But as noted above, if you're a girl with such issues, observers may think it *must* be something extraordinary, well beyond ADHD, compelling you to act this way. Even more, the inattentive symptoms of ADHD are subtle and harder to measure. Thus, progress is more difficult to detect without a fine-grained set of assessments (such as the number of problems attempted and completed in class or during homework, or the numbers of adult prompts required to main-tain performance). As for the struggle for accommodations, or the additional work needed to understand just how well medication or behavioral treatments are working, it takes time and effort to measure symptoms, impairments, and progress, especially for girls with ADHD. Again, overtly disruptive behaviors (more prevalent in boys) are easier to track, so that you, as the parent of a girl with ADHD, may need to be super-aware and super-diligent in documenting progress or falling back.

Be Aware of Female-Specific Issues and Coping Mechanisms

It's not my goal to make facile gender stereotypes. But scientific evidence, along with my own long-term work in this area, compels me to assert the fol-lowing. Many girls with ADHD are all too aware that they can't perform as easily or as productively as their agemates—even though it may take them a long time to understand that this "thing" called ADHD may lie at the core of the problem. And, like so many girls, they desperately want to fit in, to be valued by their families, to be accepted by their peers, and not to be the source of castigation and even ridicule from teachers and other school personnel. As a result, some girls with ADHD—more so than boys—*internalize* their perceived deficits and take on huge amounts of self-blame. Little wonder that rates of comorbid depression and anxiety are so high in girls with ADHD.

Others (including perhaps a large number of those with internalization tendencies) fight hard to compensate. For instance, they hyperstudy or engage in other means of defying the 24-hour daily schedule in which we all function. They feel they just have to somehow get the grade of A and/or prove to the world that they are just fine.

Recall the *triple bind* described earlier in the book. As they approach and enter their teen years, girls—including those with ADHD—are expected to perform the impossible triad of being nurturing and compassionate, behaving in truly competitive ways, and doing both in an effortless and sexualized fashion. For a girl displaying prominent symptoms of ADHD, the stress and strain can become unmanageable. In many cases, she will try to swim upstream frantically, compensating and overtrying—making it hard to detect the underlying symptoms and placing her under frightening levels of strain.

The bottom line? It may be easy to miss girls with legitimate ADHD if you look only at their performance levels. Especially in grade school, with one teacher all day and with large amounts of parental scaffolding, the symptoms may be relatively hidden. Yet what are the inner costs—particularly when the ante is raised in middle school and high school, with multiple subjects, teachers, and demands for organization and independence?

What I ask for now is for you to look honestly at your daughter and try to discern (and help others discern) what her behavior is like when either she's not in hyperdrive or you aren't overly engaged in helping her compensate. During the assessment process, for example, it's important for the evaluator to inquire as to her behavior patterns when she's not under real scrutiny from you or other adults. Ask her teacher(s) how she might perform without regular supports. Otherwise, the core issues related to ADHD may well be missed.

• • •

In summary, schools are the venues in which ADHD is often revealed to its fullest. As a parent, you must get an evidence-based evaluation of your daughter; know your rights as to mandated accommodations; and ensure that her teachers are managing problem behavior, promoting attention and academic success, and scaffolding executive functions with evidence-based treatments.

Helping Your Young Daughter with ADHD Thrive

In Chapter 6 we covered important ground on evidence-based treatments; in Chapter 7, the topic was educating your daughter with ADHD. This chapter now incorporates that information into the specifics of parenting a girl with ADHD who is in preschool or grade school. In particular, I offer tips and strategies regarding parenting (see also Chapter 5), take a deeper dive into enhancing your daughter's social relationships—at home, in school, and in the neighborhood—and cover practical issues related to medication. An additional aim is to highlight those particular factors and processes during childhood that predict difficult outcomes in adolescence and beyond, especially the display of self-harmful behaviors that are distressingly common in girls with ADHD as they grow older. In Chapter 9, I address the same topic areas but with a switch to teenagers, focusing on adolescent experiences and other factors that can contribute to negative adult outcomes. I've divided this material into two chapters to keep each at readable length but also because there are some significant differences in parenting girls at these two developmental stages. Indeed, teenage girls with ADHD raise a whole new set of issues and challenges (and potential strengths) beyond those encountered in childhood.

Your Top 10 Guidelines for Parenting Preteen Girls with ADHD

Following are some overall guidelines and strategies presented as a Top 10 list. You'll find strategies at the end of each guideline and more detailed examples and vignettes of key practices later in the chapter.

1. *Get competent professional help for assessment and treatment.* Enlisting professionals with reputations for conducting evidence-based assessments and interventions is crucial. Especially for girls in preschool or early elementary-school grades, most general pediatricians—or psychologists without deep training and experience in ADHD—may miss the boat, either overdiagnosing it (especially in boys) or underdiagnosing or calling it something else (especially in girls). It can take some real work on your part to find a professional with the chops to perform a thorough and evidence-based evaluation (see Chapter 2 for details).

Don't stop with your regular pediatrician. Get their advice on specialists and talk with other parents—perhaps via support groups—about the best referrals in your area. Don't be afraid to ask potential assessors how they approach evaluation: "How long would you expect the evaluation to take? Do you use rating scales . . . interview families carefully . . . make school observations or otherwise get direct teacher input? What additional testing would be part of the assessment?" Finally, inquire about subsequent treatment options: "Do you know professionals in the area who perform behavioral family therapy? Do you work collaboratively with them?"

2. *Get your daughter's teachers and school on board for intervention.* As emphasized in Chapter 7, enlisting teachers and school personnel is essential. Obtaining formal accommodations can be a step along this path. Yet with or without accommodations and special services, it takes considerable effort on your part—using a blend of diplomacy and assertion—to get teachers and school administrators aligned as full participants in the behavioral strategies known to work for kids with ADHD.

Rearrange your work schedule, as best you can, to meet teachers in person (or on Zoom) before or after school to "talk up" your daughter and her learning needs. Ask directly about the teacher's views on ADHD. Be as clear as you can be about what you've learned with respect to classroom strategies that work best for her. For instance: "Have you taught girls (or boys) with ADHD before? What worked best in your view? How do you structure your classroom to allow for different learning styles?" What you're shooting for here is the formation of an alliance—and getting the teacher to see your daughter's strengths as well as areas needing remediation.

3. *Make it a team effort.* Helping girls with ADHD of any age thrive is truly a group enterprise: Neither your daughter nor you can do it alone. Get

a team engaged while she is still young—relatives, friends, tutors, advocates, and after-school personnel, beyond teachers and school staff. Self-help and advocacy groups can be a real source of education and mutual problem solving, also serving as a resource for competent professionals in your area. There's no shame, and plenty to gain, in leaning on others throughout your journey.

As you accumulate advocates, consider hosting a home get-together (when your daughter is perhaps at a neighbor's), inviting relatives, sitters, friends, and/ or volunteers in her life (this could also be through a group Zoom meeting). The goal: To build enthusiasm and strategies—and to share ideas around the kinds of tactics that target her particular needs. If "live," provide food (or make it a potluck), so that people feel welcome.

4. *Maintain a positive outlook while preventing the stigmatization of your daughter and family.* Sadly, a diagnosis of ADHD can still be a source of shame and stigma. This is especially likely if your attitude, or that of your extended family, is that the label is disgraceful, signaling flaws in your daughter or your parenting approach. It can take considerable work to overcome such feelings, beliefs, and attitudes. Learning what ADHD actually entails (see the first five chapters of this book) and educating those in your world about its realities are part of the journey. Whether she lets you know it or not, your daughter is likely to "read" your own attitudes and beliefs, with the potential for internalizing negative perceptions and blaming herself. No one thrives if the overriding sense is one of shame and recrimination.

First, stigma regarding ADHD is everywhere, especially given the bad press surrounding it. Such stigmatization may reveal itself as partially masked statements like the following: "That family is just trying to get a diagnosis and accommodations for a lazy, spoiled girl." "Everyone knows that there's no such thing as ADHD." "How dare they think that their daughter needs something special from school: All kids need special attention." A calm, nondefensive, information-laden approach is a good idea here. Federal and state laws, and gradually evolving attitudes, are on your side. You can provide reminders that it wasn't so long ago that children with vision or hearing problems, or other physical disabilities, were denied services. You can also point to a whole lot of science that backs the reality of ADHD.

Second, as for your own attitudes, you might ask your partner, or friends of yours, or others who know you and your daughter, for some honest feedback about how you communicate to the world (both verbally and nonverbally) about her. Perhaps you give off the vibe that you're more ashamed of her, and/or your own parenting, than you realize or care to admit to yourself. For a refresher on the actual causes of ADHD, go back to Chapter 4.

Third, make lists of your daughter's strengths and periodically review (and update) these. Examine your own expectations for her and find ways to modify them (for example, does she just have to get all As, every term?). Recall times when you were struggling as a child and consider positive influences in your life back then. As you do all this, you may come to realize that people with ADHD have both strengths and weaknesses. Stigma and stress will diminish when you're on the side of emphasizing your daughter's positives while fighting for services and treatments that will allow her to build additional skills.

5. *Be proactive in preventing your daughter's self-blame.* Girls and boys with ADHD too often lack deep insight into their behavior patterns, have a low reserve of intrinsic motivation for routine or difficult tasks, and show a lack of real interest in becoming involved in needed treatments. As well, girls with ADHD are highly prone to develop a sense that they are unlovable (think of the frequent arguments and yelling at home) and unteachable (especially if they have been criticized by teachers or removed from classrooms because of misbehavior or poor ability to learn). Positive behavior change is the answer, at a slow and steady clip, to relieve guilt and shame. Reassuring your daughter in productive ways is a big part of the solution here.

Shame in a child may look different from shame in a teen. Younger girls may shut down, or throw a fit, or refuse to keep trying (without saying many, if any, words about it). Teens, on the other hand, are often more vocal in blaming both themselves and those close to them (like their parents!). At the same time, many parents don't want to deal with negative self-attitudes in their daughter, which are really painful to acknowledge. But it's more than OK to actively notice such perceptions and help your daughter work through them. For example:

"It must be hard, sweetie, to think that your teacher is against you. If you can keep up with your reward chart and daily report card, I'd bet that she might change how she thinks about you." Or, *"We all blame ourselves when things go wrong. You have ADHD, which makes it harder to concentrate and focus than for other girls. And we're all working to give you some steps to work on it."* Additionally, *"Did you know that athletes like Simone Biles and Michael Phelps have ADHD? And still get help for it even now?"*

6. *Use rewards and incentives—and medications when indicated.* As repeatedly emphasized in Chapter 6, effective treatment strategies for girls with ADHD involve incentive-based reward programs, plus intentional teaching to improve organizational skills and executive functions. Medication is also an important treatment, given that the primary medications for ADHD enhance motivation, produce more focus, and promote better self-restraint and inhibition.

In short, engage deeply in treatment. "Get wet all over!" a coach of mine used to say many years ago when I was a high-school athlete (and he was not a swimming coach—he was referring to going "all in" for any sport). It might feel foolish or futile to praise your daughter more than you do her siblings, or to have a visible reward chart. But the dividends can be real.

7. *Keep yourself as the focus, too.* Don't forget to prioritize yourself during the assessment and treatment process. Keep in mind that it can be a ton of work (and a real investment) to secure an evaluation and initiate treatment. Doing so may alter the status quo, and change is always hard. Still, the ultimate goal is to reduce stress and enhance skill development for the whole family, leading to lowered strain and a better life for everyone. None of this is easy; there will be growing pains as attitudes change and family members develop new skills.

Try self-talk: "Yeah, I've had to change my approach, and it's just plain hard. But the other parents in our behavioral group seem to have made progress."

"If I worry about her 24/7, how much will I have in the tank when the going gets really tough? I need to do my best in the reward program—and try to let it go if there are setbacks."

"What have we got to lose as a family? Maybe things can really improve!"

"I have to give up the sense that my daughter needs to like me all the time. If I set clearer limits, I won't end up being so negative and she will have a better chance of improving."

8. *Consider your own potential need for assessment and treatment.* It's crucial to probe your own levels of anxiety, depression, and/or ADHD. As highlighted in Chapter 6, treatment for such conditions, if they are present, can greatly assist in your ability to engage in behavioral strategies and other needed supports for your daughter. Indeed, getting treatment for yourself can have major benefits for everyone. Research reveals when parents themselves have prominent symptoms of ADHD, their improvement in such symptoms

predicts better child outcomes, linked chiefly to reductions in their negative parenting behaviors.

If there's any doubt, seek an evaluation for yourself. It's truly stressful to be the parent of a girl with ADHD—and many parents may well be experiencing similar symptoms. A good evaluation can help sort out what are your longstanding issues and what are, instead, understandable reactions to raising a daughter with ADHD. As needed, treatment should be a family affair.

Again, try self-talk: "Yeah, maybe I've been ignoring how devastated I feel for too long. If I try to sacrifice myself for her, we might all go down with the ship. I recognize that when I observe her, I see myself when I was young, even though no one thought that girls had ADHD back then. Maybe I should actually get myself evaluated."

9. *Reward your own achievements.* Take time to reward yourself as a parent, and as a family, for insights you gain, for important skills you learn during treatment, and for gradual behavior change in both you and your daughter. Adults may have greater levels of intrinsic motivation than youth, but all of us need to recognize and incentivize positive change. These points are especially true given the inevitable ups and downs, struggles, and even battles that occur when trying to make your home and school behavioral programs work effectively. If you're taking pains to reward your daughter, don't neglect yourself.

Possible self-rewards? Binge-watch your favorite TV series (OK, in moderation). Have a small celebration with your partner or with a good friend. Do extra meditation or relaxation, if that's a source of stress relief for you. Have your partner or a good friend buy you some gift cards—and use one when you see progress. Make your own reward chart, giving yourself a star (with a good backup reward, like a nice dinner) when you see progress.

10. *Stay aware of ADHD-related findings and news.* As time allows, try to read up on trends in the worlds of ADHD research and treatment. While doing so, you will become a better consumer of advice for effective intervention strategies. You can also become a source of support to other families as you develop your own expertise and confidence. Doing all this requires that you don't fall prey to the many sources of "information" claiming that ADHD is a hoax, that behavioral programs and medications are evil means of mind control, and that the latest fad diets, herbs, supplements, and more are the quick and easy answer.

See the Resources at the end of the book for sources of sound, evidence-based information.

Helping Your Preschool Daughter Thrive

The consensus is that ADHD is typically a lifelong condition, starting in childhood and usually persisting into adulthood, even though certain symptoms (like hyperactivity per se) may decrease. Levels of impairment typically wax and wane over the years, depending on contexts and situations. Still, how early can a family or professional really know whether a young child has ADHD—or at least has a real risk for developing it?

Identifying ADHD in Preschoolers: A Tricky Balancing Act

This topic is the subject of major debate. In fact, to develop self-control, all toddlers and preschoolers require adult guidance and scaffolding, plus the time, positive bonds, and proper nutrition for healthy brain development. There's a real danger in overattributing problematic levels of "the terrible twos" automatically to ADHD, when in many cases such behaviors are on the high end of the "normal" range and should taper off through maturation. Provocative new research has revealed some reliable indicators of ADHD by the toddler years, but many more studies remain to be performed in this regard before the findings are validated.

> *Diagnosing a girl with strong signs of ADHD by age 4 can head off serious problems in the years to come.*

Yet during the preschool years, and particularly by age 4, strong signs of ADHD can be diagnosed. In fact, they clearly *should* be diagnosed and treated if present, to head off serious problems in grade school and beyond. The process begins with a thorough evaluation, as emphasized in Chapter 2.

Impulsivity and Hyperactivity as Hallmark Symptoms in the Youngest Children

How does ADHD present itself during these early years? It becomes clearly noticeable at ages 4 and 5 (and perhaps even as early as age 3) when there are extremely high displays of impulsivity and hyperactivity. Certain preschoolers—more boys than girls, by a factor of over 3:1 or 4:1—stand out in preschools (and at home) because of their engagement of "in your face," overly active, and often quite disruptive behavior patterns. Many of them have been noticeable to parents from the toddler years, or even in utero, because of the high levels of motion involved. Temperamental traits of extreme activity levels, high intensity, and low degrees of effortful control can be present during the first year of life.

By preschool, many if not most children meeting criteria for ADHD fall into the designation "hyperactive-impulsive," meaning that they may not show the requisite number of inattentive symptoms (because they're not yet in formal schooling) but are instead loaded with high levels of impulsivity and hyperactivity. They stand out because teachers and parents alike cannot contain them. Some such children may even pose a real threat to agemates, or themselves, because of reckless behavior.

Whereas a number of preschoolers may be slower to develop self-control than others, I'm talking here about those 4- and 5-year-old children who are truly extreme with respect to disruptive actions, risk taking, running around, and even displays of dangerous behaviors, when contrasted with their peers. Life at home is typically quite stressful, given the disruptiveness and sheer exhaustion experienced by parents, siblings, and relatives. When preschool begins, with its demands for following directions, obeying basic rules, and participation in small and larger group interactions, the ante is raised considerably.

The official symptom lists do not well characterize how ADHD appears in preschool settings (or at home). Here are some more graphic examples:

- Constant talking and interrupting (here's a place where a girl with early-appearing ADHD may be particularly salient, even if she isn't always as physically active as young boys with ADHD are)
- Swearing or otherwise impulsively using words that are not often heard from kids at this age level
- Climbing on objects, when climbing isn't part of the routine (for example, indoors)
- Making loud and potentially inappropriate noises
- Showing frequently changing moods—it's as though whatever is now salient captures the child's full attention, with what happened even a minute or two ago seemingly gone with the wind

- Inability to sit still for even a few minutes at meals or when being read a story
- Propensity for accidental injury, because of fearless or daring behavior patterns
- Intrusive and even aggressive interactions with agemates
- Inability to wait for almost anything
- Relatedly, trouble taking turns (for example, needs to be first and/or appears to need to be the sole focus of attention)
- Near-constant fidgeting and/or being in motion (note that a longstanding item on some ADHD rating scales is "acts as if driven by a motor"). Again, many preschool girls with ADHD display this pattern of behavior, though there may be more hypertalkativeness than hyperactivity per se.

As a result, lots of areas in life are extremely challenging. For example, bedtimes can be disastrous, as the young child with ADHD just can't seem to settle and appears to need less sleep than other kids (certainly less than do adults in the home!). Exhaustion levels compound for everyone. Additionally, such activities as mealtimes, leisure time, traveling to see friends or relatives, or play periods—which, after all, are supposed to be fun—too often end up as simply frustrating, stress-laden, and exhausting.

But what about the symptoms of disorganization and poor focus, related to the inattentive form of ADHD? Are there certain children, particularly girls, whose extreme inattentiveness would be sufficiently apparent in preschool to warrant diagnosis? Here are some examples.

- Is your daughter so distractible in the preschool classroom that she can't track what the teacher is saying or other kids are doing?
- Does she appear, too often, "in a cloud"—or in her own world? (This is not the same as the aloneness or aloofness of a girl with autism spectrum disorder, but rather seems to be the result of being unable to focus without a ton of structure.)
- Are there major difficulties in following any direction of two or more parts or steps?
- Does she seem to forget the classroom routine, even though it has been repeated many times?

- Even though she may not be impulsive behaviorally (for example, inter-rupting others, performing daring behaviors), does she often say the first thing that comes to mind without giving it any apparent thought? This is a kind of "cognitive impulsivity" often associated with inatten-tive ADHD.

- Can she stay focused during circle time for only a couple of minutes?

Certainly, such extremes do exist, but it's far more difficult to detect ADHD–Inattentive in girls (or boys) during the preschool years than it is the bothersome, exhausting, and potentially dangerous behavior patterns that per-tain to the more impulsive forms of ADHD. Although being inattentive can yield strain at home and in class during these years, it is not nearly as pro-vocative as being rash and disruptive. And, until academic demands multiply in kindergarten and grade school, we tend not to think of young children as deficient in attention because the expectations revolve around play and cre-ativity as opposed to sitting still and learning preacademic or early academic material. Even though increasing pressures are now in place for pre-reading skills and attentional control ever earlier in development, inattentiveness per se is not as noticeable to preschool teachers as are oppositional and disruptive behavior patterns.

Finally, if extreme inattention—of the forms just noted—is present in girls, many teachers and even clinicians will often attribute it to anxiety, learn-ing disorders, or even sensory problems. Of course, sometimes such issues can occur in tandem with early ADHD. Overall, stereotypes still exist that ADHD is not a "girl thing," especially in the earliest years of development. The behav-iors just don't fit the stereotypes related to girls' behaviors.

In sum, if your daughter shows, at early ages, true extremes of disruptive, intrusive, uncooperative, and even dangerous behavior, it's time to get an eval-uation before she's tossed out of preschool programs and before her subsequent learning and her ability to develop better self-control are further compromised. Remember that IEPs can begin as young as age 3, although stringent documen-tation will be required. On the other hand, girls at significant risk for ADHD related to poor attention and deficient rule following, along with high levels of distractibility and poor intrinsic motivation, will usually *not* show symptoms in the diagnosable range until kindergarten or beyond, when schooling becomes more formal and structured in the early grades. Indeed, such girls may be

> *Symptoms of the inattentive presentation usually have to be extreme for ADHD to be diagnosed before kindergarten, when formal schooling is more likely to reveal a problem.*

perceived as a kind of relief, as they are not typically bothersome to others. Overall, it would take utter extremes of poor direction-following, disorganization, distractibility, and lack of follow-through to qualify for a diagnosis during the preschool years.

A Tough Adjustment

The letter from the preschool director couldn't have been clearer: Carrie had been expelled from the program. The reasons given were not completely unknown to her mom, Sandra: Frequent parent–teacher meetings had raised issues about her daughter's dangerous behaviors with other children, like pushing them when they wouldn't share with her, and her inability to follow even basic classroom rules.

Devastated, Sandra finally realized that it was time to take up the advice of relatives and friends and get Carrie evaluated by the clinical psychologist whose number Sandra had been keeping for months but could never bring herself to call. It took a while, but finally the first appointment came around, and she brought with her all of the documentation and notes of Carrie's earliest years of life, sitting with the psychologist for an hour-long interview about infancy and toddlerhood—as well as the family's ongoing stress and battles with their now 4-year-old.

Sandra completed rating scales, as did last year's preschool teacher and (grudgingly) this year's, before the expulsion. When the diagnosis of ADHD emerged, Sandra was stunned, especially with the recommendation to consider medication. Still, she decided to start a behavioral family therapy group as soon as she could.

The hard work—going back to the school district to get an IEP, finding a preschool with a bit more tolerance for girls with behavioral and attentional challenges, and forging a basic DRC with the preschool—gave Sandra some confidence that her daughter would complete her second year of preschool with a real chance at succeeding in kindergarten. In fact, a huge part of this was building into her accommodations a part-time aide for the preschool classroom, not simply to shadow Carrie but to give the head teacher another set of eyes and ears, to provide both Carrie and her peers some individualized attention.

In fact, with kindergarten looming, Sandra has engaged the developmental/behavioral pediatrician (referred by the clinical psychologist) in active discussions about a medication trial. And she's begun to realize that it would take a different level of stretching herself as a parent to handle Carrie's intense style and maintain a positive bond with her.

Many parents of preschoolers with ADHD may need to "hit bottom" in this kind of way. Although painful, it can lead to the revelation that their daughter's active style and defiance were never ideal, motivating the family to get deeply engaged in treatment.

Behavioral Family Therapy

If your daughter does qualify for a diagnosis of ADHD during this period, it is essential that you engage in intensive behavioral family therapy. Even in the United States, where for older children medication is often still viewed as the primary treatment modality, behavioral family interventions are the clear first intervention choice for preschoolers with ADHD. It's also crucial that home–school efforts be coordinated. As noted below, medications have real limitations for preschool children with ADHD, showing relatively small effects in many cases, with increased chances for side effects compared to older children. Taking major steps to alter home and preschool contexts—and to provide clear expectations and frequent rewards—is the treatment of choice.

As discussed in Chapter 6, most kids with ADHD, both boys and girls, require external structure and extrinsic rewards to motivate positive behaviors—and this is much more the case for preschoolers. Simple and clear directions, concrete rewards (and easy-to-follow reward charts), and joint work with the preschool teacher are all crucial. Equally important is your understanding that *now* is the time to get serious about your daughter's problems.

School districts may resist any notion that a preschool-age girl can really have an ADHD diagnosis, so I encourage you to find the best diagnosticians available when you're seeing clear signs of ADHD, even if your daughter's teacher believes that it must be some other problem or issue. Gaining accommodations for your daughter at this stage of development is no easy matter, but if her behavior patterns are sufficiently severe, the earlier you can engage in home and school behavioral interventions, the better.

Let me say it a different way: If your daughter is in the diagnostic range for ADHD by age 4 or 5, with behavioral patterns that might derail her for years to come, it is *not* a good idea to simply wait and see. I'm referring to physically dangerous behaviors, oppositionality that has thwarted most if not all family harmony, and expulsion (or threats thereof) from preschool. In such cases, the chances for the continuation of behavioral, cognitive, and emotional problems are strong unless intervention is started. Yet if the situation is not urgent and if clear impairment is not present, it could be wise to wait until kindergarten and see what emerges—while still adding as many supports for your daughter and yourself as possible.

What might a home reward program look like for a preschool-age girl with ADHD? Let's start with what it would *not* look like: a large and complicated chart with many rows of target behaviors and columns of point totals. Young girls with ADHD need something immediate, tangible, and eye-catching. Consider a set of smaller charts—one of them with 2 key mealtime targets (for example, staying seated from setting the timer until it sounds; talking in a soft voice), another with a bedtime target (listening calmly during bedtime story), another with a morning target (getting dressed with some assistance without a tantrum), and the like. Make the stars for attaining the targets visible, and always accompany the awarding of stars or points with real praise and enthusiasm. At the same time, DRCs should be simple and easy for your daughter to track.

The core aim is to reverse the contingencies in many homes of young kids with ADHD, where the majority of a parent's words to their child are reminders, scolds, criticisms, or threats. Aim to make it a 5:1 ratio (or more) of positive statements to negative ones!

How to talk with your daughter after misbehavior? Despite the best-planned reward charts, with attainable target behaviors at the outset, your daughter will of course not always succeed.

Don't: Yell, berate, or remind her angrily that she's ruined the day yet again. The calmer you remain, the better, as you won't be responding to failed attempts or frank problem behavior with attention (even negative attention is *some* kind of attention for her).

Do: Let her know that she has not earned her star, model what she needs to do, and give her an opportunity as soon as practicable to try again.

How to pace yourself in implementing a reward program for your exhausting daughter? First, do not expect overnight miracles. She has been dealing with the temperament she was born with for several years now, and the whole family may be accustomed to a routine of overtiredness, begging, yelling, and paying far more attention to her misbehavior than to her positive behavior. Second, set reasonable and attainable goals, based on the charting of her behavior. Third, realize that you can't be her companion, teacher, and behavioral coach 24/7. Have other family members take over responsibility, when possible, and realize that some other things in your life (for example, a perfectly clean house all the time) may just have to slide as you gear up your program.

A note on kindergarten: I highlight a research finding that has gained a lot of attention in recent years. Specifically, children who start kindergarten at age 4 (because they happen to have been born just before the district's kindergarten-entry cutoff age, such as September 1) as opposed to age 5 (because they happen to have been born just after the cutoff) are much more likely to be diagnosed with ADHD by the end of kindergarten. The implication is that young and potentially immature 4-year-olds can get misdiagnosed with ADHD. This is an intriguing and potentially troubling issue, which I could discuss at length. But the point I wish to make is that in the largest study of this issue to date, the finding was clear-cut for boys but not nearly as strong (and not "statistically significant") for girls. Nonetheless, during kindergarten, if you or the teacher begin to suspect ADHD, make sure that the assessment and diagnostic process is thorough, complete, and evidence-based. There are a lot of issues in young children (for example, response to maltreatment, medical conditions, serious anxiety) that appear similar to ADHD but require differential diagnosis.

> *Starting kindergarten at age 4 may lead to a (sometimes mistaken) diagnosis of ADHD by the end of the school year because immaturity can be misinterpreted as ADHD symptoms.*

Behavioral Family Strategies in Action

Amanda and Jose's 4-year-old daughter, Jessie, has always seemed to be a challenge. Amanda can vouch that Jessie was on the move even during pregnancy. As an infant, Jessie was super-intense, with real difficulties settling into any routines. When Jessie was a toddler, Amanda and Jose "childproofed" their home environment but need to do so even now. They hesitated to put Jessie in preschool, but life at home has been laden with frustration and exhaustion. A friend, the parent of a girl with ADHD, got them a referral to see a behavioral specialist. Here are some of the things that the parents are now trying.

Directions: *"Jessie, look right at me. Excellent. Now listen—put away your toys, now." This kind of basic direction is what the parents had to give to their first child when he was 2, but they had learned that they must use the same slow and methodical procedures with Jessie, even at age 4.*

Praise: *After another prompt, Amanda says, "Great, Jessie, thanks for putting your toys back. Here's a star on your chart." It seems so basic, but this is what it takes for a girl with ADHD, Amanda has learned.*

After rule breaking: *"Jessie, no hitting your brother. That's a time-out. Come to your chair." Jose has stopped yelling at Jessie when she hits her brother and has now learned to calmly enforce a 2-minute time-out.*

Don't: *Engage in the following. "How many times will it take for you to learn not to hit your brother? Just STOP it before I scream." (Note: You're already screaming.)*

Do: *In a calm tone, say, "That's hitting, so it's a time-out. Come to your chair now." (Note: For really defiant young children with ADHD who refuse to go to time-out, there are resources at the end of the book, as in the* Defiant Children *program of Russell Barkley.)*

Amanda and Jose have begun to structure their daughter's environment according to her developmental level (which is actually closer to age 2 than age 4), while maintaining a positive and supportive tone. Chapter 5 emphasized that authoritative parenting is a great blend of warmth/responsiveness and structure/limit setting; this is precisely what the parents are now striving to enact. Although time-out procedures have been criticized (with the assumption that they might disrupt attachment if your child is isolated in a time-out chair), research reveals that they can actually promote better bonding—far more so than physical punishments—if done calmly and clearly and when you reengage your daughter in the home's activities as the time-out ends.

Social Skills and Peer Relationships

One of the huge risks of preschool-age ADHD is that your daughter will be rejected by her peers. This is likely for girls with ADHD even more than for boys with ADHD, as girls place a particularly high premium on smooth and cooperative social interactions. A girl showing rampant ADHD behavior patterns can threaten social harmony: Her impulsive and intrusive behaviors may make her seem to be a bully at worst—or at least insensitive to the needs of her peers, not a good choice as a playmate. Peer relationships begin in earnest during early childhood, and a girl with early ADHD will inadvertently push peers away via impulsive, aggressive, and self-centered behavior patterns. Poor reading of the social cues of girls in her classroom and neighborhood is another culprit here. Importantly, it may be difficult for her to regain peer supports as she later begins formal schooling, because peer rejection is tantamount to being "expelled" from playdates, birthday parties, or outings. If peers have pushed her out of their circles, it's going to be really hard to learn effective social skills. What can you do?

1. Make sure that your home (and preschool) reward program includes peer interactions, including limits on aggressive behaviors and ample, immediate rewards for positive social encounters.

2. Encourage playdates. In some cases you may need to solicit parents of agemates to give it a try—and to supervise these encounters more than would be usual.

3. Model for your daughter calm interactions, devoid of yelling and arguments, as the template for how people treat other people. For example, you can role-play sharing and turn taking with her. You can also point out positive social behaviors demonstrated in books or on television, reviewing those with her. Behaviorally oriented social skills groups for older girls with ADHD offer just this kind of explicit modeling, guidance, feedback, and reward.

4. Provide support and consolation when your daughter expresses sadness over a lack of playmates or friends. Let her know that she remains a good person, worthy of attention and love—and that she can practice becoming a better friend.

5. Realize that as your daughter gains better self-regulation, there will be chances for positive peer encounters, as long as she receives more-than-typical levels of support, guidance, praise, and tangible rewards as early as you can offer them. Of course, you can't come in and totally take over unfolding interactions your daughter has on a playdate or on the preschool playground. But you can work with the other key adults in her life to model, encourage, and provide direct feedback for building blocks of social interactions.

> *Creating an environment for your daughter to build social skills early can help to head off years of painful rejection by peers.*

Medications

What about stimulant medication, or other medications for ADHD, with respect to preschool-age girls with the diagnosis? The initial multicenter study of medication treatments for preschoolers with ADHD—both boys and girls—revealed that stimulant medications can and do help with reduction of relevant symptoms. Yet overall effects were not as large as those with older children. Around half of preschoolers with ADHD showed a positive medication response, compared to three-quarters or more of older kids. Even more, medications yielded a greater chance of side effects for young children than they did for older kids (for example, appetite disturbances, sleep issues, irritability, explosive behavior). Therefore, if medications are tried, official guidelines recommend beginning with low dosage levels—and with the methylphenidate class of stimulants as the first to be tried, before amphetamine-style stimulants. The reason is that there are more studies of methylphenidate-style meds with preschoolers. As well, amphetamines are more "potent," milligram per milligram, than the methylphenidate group. This can usually be worked around by simply giving half the dosage of an amphetamine, but such practice is not always followed.

As noted, official U.S. guidelines recommend that behavior therapy approaches are the first line of treatment for preschoolers with ADHD. This recommendation does *not* mean that you should never consider medications for preschool-age girls with ADHD. A medication trial could well be indicated if family and school behavior therapy has not been successful. It may also be in order for cases marked by behavioral extremes. In fact, well-delivered medications can make the difference between remaining in preschool and leaving, or between a reasonably calm home life and one marked by extreme stress, separation, or even maltreatment. It can also be essential for young children with severe ADHD who may not be safe because of dangerous behaviors related to themselves or others. Indeed, preschool-age children with ADHD, including girls, are at high risk for serious physical injuries and emergency department visits, linked to impulsive and risk-taking behaviors (for example, jumping or falling from high places, running into the street). Still, medications require supplementation with intentional, structured, and well-delivered home- and school behavioral therapy interventions for preschoolers. A full-on team effort is required.

Finally, many parents of preschoolers suspected of having ADHD, or recently diagnosed with ADHD, are frankly afraid of the thought that their child might receive stimulant medication, often portrayed as monstrous means of chemical control of the behaviors of innocent youngsters. Without the space to engage in a long debate here, I offer three points.

1. The decision to begin medication is a serious one, requiring consultation with a trusted doctor who is experienced with medicating young children with ADHD.

2. For the reasons listed just above, in some cases preschoolers with severe ADHD may well require medications to supplement behavioral programs.

3. Performing a trial of ADHD medications is not a lifetime commitment. Because most ADHD medications have short half-lives, their effects can usually be observed relatively quickly, not requiring periods of many weeks or months (which can often be the case for many other types of psychiatric medications).

Please remember from Chapter 6 that it may take trying several different kinds of medication, and/or dosage levels, before you know whether there's a positive response. Whether the trial is successful or not, the information you gain can be important for you, your daughter, and your family. In short, engaging in a well-delivered medication trial may provide answers, but you will need to let go of the scare tactics involved in lots of anti-ADHD and anti-medication rhetoric.

Medications such as guanfacine and clonidine may be the best choice for the youngest girls with ADHD because they cause fewer side effects than stimulants. But you won't know without a medication trial.

Please note: A recent, large study revealed information on the alpha-2, norepinephrine-targeted medications (for example, guanfacine, clonidine) for preschoolers. In brief, they showed fewer side effects than stimulants for preschool-age children. As a result, these could well be a consideration if your preschool-age daughter displays ADHD.

The Elementary Years

Referrals to clinicians for diagnoses of ADHD spike during grade school. Boys tend to have peak referrals in second through fourth grade, once elementary-school teachers, often to their dismay, notice the impulsive and disruptive behavior patterns that can wreak havoc on lesson plans and classroom routines. These years are also a period of high referral rates for girls with prominent impulsivity and hyperactivity, linked to the combined presentation of ADHD. But for those girls with inattention and poor executive functions as the primary area of concern, it may not be until late elementary school, middle school, or even high school that clinical concerns regarding ADHD arise. As emphasized throughout this book, parents, teachers, and clinicians may not believe that ADHD actually occurs in girls—and even if they do, they may well overlook ADHD in females because a "spacy" style, lack of organization, and overtalkativeness don't seem to fit the ADHD mold, which still prioritizes boys. At the same time, girls may keep their heads (barely) above water in elementary school as long as families provide huge supports—and the girls themselves compensate with supreme effort to overcome underlying disorganization and poor self-control. Although core symptoms may be masked, strong risk for anxiety, worries, reduced self-esteem, and peer problems can multiply. In short, the elementary grades are a key period during which many girls with ADHD first show symptoms.

> *Girls who show ADHD symptoms at home but are (barely) getting by at school should not be left untreated, because their risk for anxiety, low self-esteem, and peer problems is likely to grow while their symptoms go unaddressed.*

Working Collaboratively with a Teacher

Jasmine's teacher sent a note to her parents via e-mail. It said that the DRC he had initiated for their fifth-grade daughter was falling apart. That is, he said, Jasmine was getting too many no responses for the targets of ignoring rather than teasing other peers if she was teased, turning in work on time, and staying organized during transitions from one subject to another. Jasmine's mom had noticed this pattern of increasing nos herself, but now the teacher was clearly concerned.

And this was the year prior to the dreaded start of middle school! Fighting panic, Mom sucked it up and asked for a Zoom call after school when the teacher's schedule was free. She feared that this teacher, whom both parents believed really did have their daughter's best interests at heart, still may not "get it" that there's such a thing as the inattentive form of ADHD. He had seemed initially reluctant to go along with the DRC, and now in its fourth week, the program seemed to be tanking.

During the call, Mom strained to remember what their behavior therapist had told them as they set up the DRC. "If there are not enough yes responses coming back home," she said, "make the target behaviors more specific and a bit simpler." Patiently, they tried to let the teacher know that they appreciated his support. Yet before they launched into making the target behaviors easier to fulfill, Mom found it in herself to ask an inspired question: "What are the moments each day when you find Jasmine at her best?"

This question led to an unexpected direction. The teacher discussed what a leader Jasmine was when she was asked to talk, in class, about her painting and drawing. "If only," he continued, "she could be this interested in her core subjects."

All of a sudden, Mom and the teacher found themselves in a different kind of conversation. (1) The teacher followed the plan to ease off on the expectation for the number of pages of schoolwork, making the yes response easier to attain for the time being. (2) He also made sure that there was a way to ensure that the homework was done the previous night via the school district's online grading system. This process prevented Jasmine from forgetting to turn the assignment in on her own. (3) Most important, he worked with Mom to find rewards during the school day that had to do with extra time for Jasmine's art projects and having her help other girls with their own art. Suddenly, a positive vibe replaced the negative, even punitive tone.

Within a few weeks, Jasmine's DRC yes responses from school were way up. Her parents sensed that the teacher understood their daughter better, and both parents had become prouder of Jasmine's inherent talents in art and of her increased focus on other subjects.

Here the parents worked super-hard with the teacher to keep the DRC program alive. They also started to "bend" a bit—in other words, they began to understand that their daughter really was talented at art and that, in the future, this could become a real avenue for her. Maybe she would never be the world's best scientist, but they could utilize her interest in art to motivate better skill levels and performance in more traditional school sub-jects. In other words, recalling Chapter 5, they found a wider sense of "fit" for Jasmine—adapting some of their expectations to match her talents.

Of course, this also meant they had found different ways of connecting with and appreciating their daughter, still upholding the expectation that she meet her other school demands. All this contains the essence of the warmth and limits of authoritative parenting. Caregiving any youth requires a lot of give and take, especially when you have a daughter with ADHD.

Behavioral Family Therapy

Positive expectations, delivery of clear and direct instructions, reward charts, clear negative contingencies, home–school coordination and daily report cards, assisting in the promotion of executive functions and academic foundations—all of these are of primary importance in helping to nurture, manage, and assist your daughter with ADHD during the elementary-school years. Chapter 6 covered these points, but I will try to get down to ground level to bring home some of the most crucial ones. Below, I spend the most time on parenting stress because I believe that it is of central importance to raising a daughter with ADHD.

Parenting Stress

For parents like you, with histories of encountering ADHD in your daughter, it's quite common to experience a high degree of parenting stress, intermixed with self-recrimination and even shame. There are many mean-ings of the often-used term *stress;* here I'm referring to a mismatch between the demands of a situation (providing an optimal home environment for a girl with ADHD) and the resources available to you, both internal and external ("I wasn't prepared for this—and feel defeated . . . where can I turn for help?"). Signs of parenting stress can be as follows:

- Why isn't she thriving, the way the daughters of my friends or other families seem to be? I must be doing something wrong.
- Is it really possible that she's lost her homework for the third time this week? Come on!
- How dare she challenge my authority—I'm her parent!
- Maybe she has a hearing problem? I mean, I keep reminding her, as gently as I can at first, what she needs to do, but she just can't seem to

follow even a basic two-part direction. I get so frustrated that I could scream.

- I seem to be a constant nag, and it just creates more conflict between us: *Straighten up your room; it's a pig sty in there! We're late for school, again! Don't talk back to me that way! Homework NOW—or else. OK, OK, have it your way—just no more arguing, all right?* And I feel worse and worse each time I yell or finally give in.

- Why do so few girls invite her to get-togethers, parties, or events? Does she really not get it about give-and-take with other kids? I must have failed as a parent.

- Even on the best days, when I've made every attempt to be supportive, we both end up feeling defeated.

- Things are at such a point of frustration and conflict that I don't see how I can ever effectively parent her.

- Any closeness we used to have seems to be vanishing. And the whole family is feeling the strain.

In other words, parenting stress signifies a lack of perceived ability to perform the parenting role, a chronic feeling of being overwhelmed, a sense of poor bonding with your daughter, considerable frustration, and all too often a large amount of self-blame. It can fuel a vicious cycle of recrimination, increasing distance between you and your daughter, and promoting her internalized sense that she must be a failure—a disappointment to you and to herself. As noted earlier, my research team has found that particularly for families of girls with ADHD, high degrees of parenting stress are common. Even more, such stress is predictive of young-adult negative outcomes, like your daughter's propensity for depression and engagement in NSSI.

> *New ways of interacting, taught in behavioral family therapy, not only help your daughter thrive but can also reduce your stress tremendously.*

The crucial aim of behavioral family therapy is to engage in a new regimen of clear expectations, the positive frame that your grade-school-age daughter can and will learn better behaviors and skills through a structured reward program, clear limits that are enforced nonemotionally, collaboration with her school, and gradually enhancing her intrinsic motivation.

Lowering Stress for Mother and Daughter

It's homework time for third-grade Melissa, and she yet again gets up from her desk after a few minutes, frustration written all over her face and permeating her body language. She complains that the problems are too hard and that she just can't stand this any longer. Why put her through this torture? Her mother, Laura, fears that a meltdown or tantrum will soon follow.

Yet now that they've been through a number of sessions of behavioral family therapy, Laura reminds herself not to yell, or nag, but instead to point to the reward chart near her chair.

"Honey, look, I know this is hard. But look, I forgot to start the timer! My mistake. Remember what we talked about at the beginning of the week? If you can work for 10 minutes in a row, the 'check' on your chart can earn you extra time taking care of our pet. Let's try a little deep breathing and try again."

The reminder and the breathing exercises calm Melissa down a bit, and Laura sets the timer on the side of her desk. "Remember, 10 minutes and you get that checkmark on your chart."

"OK," Melissa says warily, "can I really have extra time with the dog if I do this?"

"Yes," Laura reminds her, "and think of those yeses that came home from your teacher today on your daily report card. These are starting to add up.

"Let's start," Laura adds as she sets the timer.

Laura didn't give undue attention to the forthcoming emotional explosion but instead calmly redirected her daughter. She also kept the tone positive—even reminding Melissa of success with the teacher-completed DRC. Crucially, she kept to the limit of holding her accountable for 10 minutes of performance (up from 8 minutes the week before—embracing small steps toward success is the way to go).

In other words, Laura showed the key elements of authoritative parenting: warmth and responsiveness intermixed with clear limits (not harsh, but not caving in either). At the same time, she encouraged her daughter's increasing independence, another key part of authoritative parenting. In fact, by calmly admitting her mistake in failing to set the timer, she also modeled the back-and-forth exchanges and the reasoning that are characteristic of an authoritative approach. Finally, the tone of the interchange was laden with a sense of connection between mother and daughter—promoting a positive bond.

Of course, it will take many more interactions like this before Laura finally senses that her family and her daughter are "getting someplace." As that goal is attained, she should experience a decrease in parenting stress. Still, she may well recall that afternoon with the forgotten timer as a signal that she finally needed to do what seemed impossible: to be warm and supportive with her daughter at the same time that she set clearer and firmer limits. The process isn't easy or linear, but once the bond becomes stronger, it can feel like more of a positive cycle.

The Home Reward Chart

As you review the principles and strategies of Chapter 6 with respect to setting up and maintaining your home reward chart, here are some prime tips for grade-school-age girls:

- Make sure that your daughter has real input into the rewards on the chart—and have a variety of such rewards, from small (redeemable on a daily basis) to intermediate (she might save up for these for a week) and then longer-term (for later elementary-age girls, stars or points that can be saved up for a special, larger reward).

Hold a conversation with your daughter about the things she likes to do and the privileges she desires. Make lists of smaller items or activities, to medium-sized ones, to larger ones that require her to save points or stars for a week or more. Get her engaged in building and filling in the reward chart.

- Ensure that the target behaviors are neither too basic nor too advanced. Your daughter needs to succeed regularly. As she does, progressively make the target goals more difficult, to build her skills. But make sure that there are initial successes.

Look at the number of points and stars, examining whether she's had those initial successes. If she's "acing" it daily, it's time to move up to more difficult targets. If she's never getting the medium or larger rewards for which she's saving, scale back the target behavior and provide additional structure and encouragement.

- When your daughter goes into a negative behavioral spiral, do your best *not* to scold or resort to yelling and screaming. All of these responses both model the kinds of behaviors that you do not want to encourage in her and may actually serve to give her a lot of attention (even if negative attention) for misbehavior. If you've clearly explained the consequences ahead of time, so that she's not taken by surprise, then the limit—when delivered clearly and calmly—serves as a signal that, to receive your positive attention and gain the reward on the chart, she will need to try again next time.

Don't: Cajole ("How many times have I told you not to tease the cat?!"), scream ("THAT'S IT—I'VE HAD IT"), bargain ("We'll let the points slide today"), or criticize/character assassinate ("How much calmer would this house be if you could only pull your act together?!").

Do: Remind gently that there are more chances; go over the chart another day when everyone is calm; be as encouraging as possible. Your ultimate aim is to work toward building a more positive and constructive relationship and home climate.

Doing all this can gradually increase your parenting confidence and reduce the awful burden of parenting stress.

Your Own ADHD, Depression, or Anxiety

As emphasized in Chapter 6, some newer, effective behavioral family therapy programs deal explicitly with the *parent's* indicators of ADHD—or significant depression and/or anxiety—to help the parent become a more positive and effective behavior manager. If these psychological issues are longstanding and/or deep-seated, they may require separate one-on-one therapy, or even medication, for you as a parent.

Communication and Coordination with School

At the risk of sounding like a broken record, I emphasize once more that when, and only when, the home and school aspects of your behavioral program are well aligned are you likely to see important changes in your daughter's academic and behavioral performance (as well as her social skills, as noted below). The DRC, featured in Chapter 7, is a mainstay of such efforts. Implementing a DRC mandates that parents, teachers, and other school personnel meet up to decide on target behaviors, make sure that the initial goals are reasonable, exchange feedback each afternoon back home, and add *yes* responses (or points) at school to your daughter's home reward system. It's simple in concept, yet it takes some work to coordinate. Importantly, it can lead to real improvements in your daughter.

The DRC and the reward chart at home are effective means of monitoring your daughter's progress. As she gains skills and reduces problem behavior, it will be time to "up" the bar of what's required over the next weeks. But if she isn't making the grade, perhaps the skills and/or problem behaviors are initially too ambitious. Break them into smaller steps and perhaps praise her efforts more frequently.

Rewarding Yourself

As noted in the Top 10 list at the beginning of this chapter, it's really important to provide yourself some positive feedback as you enter and proceed through the hard work of engaging in family behavioral therapy. Progress may be slow initially, and setbacks are inevitable. Treat yourself (and your partner, if you have one) to something special to recognize the efforts.

Social Skills and Peer Relationships

The elementary-school years are crucial for not only attaining basic academic competencies but also learning and practicing social skills with peers. Yet girls with ADHD–Combined are all too likely to be actively rejected by their age-mates, who just can't tolerate their intrusive, interruption-laden, and seemingly self-centered style. Girls with ADHD–Inattentive are often "neglected" by classmates and other peers. That is, such girls' tendencies to be daydreamy and scattered—and their potential for misreading other girls' facial cues or body language—can lead their peers to overlook them. In both cases, girls with ADHD will miss out on the very kinds of social interactions that are crucial for boosting their interpersonal abilities. For sure, this is a clear example of a vicious cycle.

For these reasons, social skills groups have been developed and researched for girls (and boys) with ADHD (see Chapter 6). The aim is for well-trained group leaders to help the kids in question learn basic facets of social interactions, via modeling, coaching, practicing, providing feedback, and rewarding increasing skill levels. What are some of these basic skills?

- Introducing yourself
- Starting and maintaining a conversation
- Speaking in a normal tone of voice rather than an overly loud manner
- Communicating reciprocally (for example, actively listening, asking about the peer's ideas or feelings, taking turns)

- Showing interest in the peer via eye contact and nonverbal behaviors like nodding
- Sharing—of toys, materials, interests
- Acknowledging, negotiating, and resolving conflicts

Social skills groups require a large amount of structure. The participants must receive rewards for basic attention to the group leaders who define and model the skills in question—and for concentrated attempts to practice as well as for overcoming mistakes and trying again. In other words, the groups need to emphasize rehearsal, not just rote learning of social skills in the abstract.

But it's not just about professionally led social skills groups. Parents—and teachers—can model, encourage, and reward gradual improvements in the kinds of important skill areas just listed. Doing so requires patience and the real sense that practice can eventually make perfect. In fact, Amori Mikami of the University of British Columbia has pioneered a program called Parental Friendship Coaching for parents of grade-school-age children with ADHD, in which parents themselves learn to model good social interactions and directly coach their daughters (and sons) in them, provide feedback, help the child select peers for playdates, and debrief with the child afterward. For more information on this program, see the Further Reading section for this chapter.

The ultimate goal is not necessarily to have your daughter with ADHD become the most popular girl in her classroom. In fact—and this is a crucial point—considerable research reveals that even a single, high-quality friendship can outweigh the consequences of being rejected or ignored by other girls. Intensive and structured social skills interventions, based on rehearsal, as well as friendship coaching, can be effective.

In short, overall positive peer regard is great, but what matters more is to have one girl (and/or a small number of peers)—whom she likes and who in turn likes her—support her, model social skills for her, and provide a base from which she gains self-esteem and a sense that she is worthwhile.

Along these lines, it may well be an important goal for you to build in accommodations to your daughter's IEP or 504 plan for her teacher to help create an "ADHD-friendly" setting.

> *Your daughter doesn't have to become the most popular girl in her class. Research shows that one good-quality friendship can work wonders.*

Indeed, all girls tend to look to their teacher when forming social preferences about their peers. The teacher's warmth, patience, acceptance, and gentle redirection of a student with ADHD can positively affect your daughter's social status. Even more, if your daughter has experienced classroom failures, it's important for the teacher to actively discover ways to draw positive attention to her. For example, the teacher could assign her tasks and responsibilities in the presence of her classmates. The aim, again, is to develop a positive view of your daughter, staving off the process of peer rejection.

Overall, for good synopses, see *https://additudemag.com/developing-social-skills* and *www.verywellmind.com/how-to-improve-social-skills-in-children-with-adhd-20727*.

Medications

In the United States, around two-thirds of youth diagnosed with ADHD are prescribed medication for their condition, which is a higher percentage than for receipt of behavioral family therapy. Unlike many other countries, several official treatment guidelines in the United States emphasize medication as the treatment of first choice for those beyond the preschool years—even though, for youth with "complex" ADHD, including comorbidities and/or substantial impairment, it's psychosocial interventions, including behavioral family therapy, that are listed as the interventions of first choice. As highlighted in Chapter 6, the best chances of promoting gains in your daughter with ADHD, beyond symptom reduction per se, emanate from the combination of well-delivered medication and behavioral therapy approaches.

Childhood is the time when medications are often initiated (although for girls, who tend to get diagnosed somewhat later than boys, it may be in adolescence or beyond when medication is first prescribed). Here are some key pointers for successful treatment of girls with ADHD through medication.

• The first type of ADHD medication your daughter tries—or the initial dose of that particular medication—may not provide optimal benefit. As well, significant side effects could emerge. It takes patience with a trial-and-error approach to make sure that she's on (1) the lowest dose possible (2) of the type of medication that works optimally for her. If I could predict, as a scientist, from an analysis of your daughter's (or anyone else's) DNA, the exact medication that would work best and at which dosage level, I would soon retire with a major scientific prize and a huge fortune. The science has simply not yet reached the stage of such precision medicine.

● Relatedly, the best way of knowing which medication and which dosage are most effective is to provide ratings, at least twice a week, on a form that includes (1) brief ADHD symptom scales, (2) other key target behaviors, and (3) potential side effects. In other words, with a standard ADHD symptom scale, you can simply add several rows, "writing in" several specific items for your daughter's own targets and a couple of common side effects. Ask her teacher to do the same. In that way, guesswork can be largely removed from the equation: You can let the numbers tell you what's working optimally. Girls with the inattentive presentation of ADHD do not, by definition, display the kinds of disruptive and easily noticeable behavior problems of their peers with high levels of impulsivity and hyperactivity. As a result, more subtle changes in direction following, attentional skills, and forgetfulness are often harder to notice. It's all the more important, therefore, to keep careful records of behavior patterns, both on and off medication and at different medication dosages. In fact, as noted in Chapter 6, youth with ADHD–Inattentive tend to require lower dosage levels than their more rambunctious counterparts. It can be easy to overmedicate them and assume that they simply are not positive medication responders because of side effects.

● In addition, girls with ADHD are slightly more likely than boys with ADHD to do well with nonstimulant medications, especially those that focus on norepinephrine as opposed to dopamine (these are the SNRIs and the alpha-2 medicines).

● If your daughter has significant comorbid disorders, like serious anxiety or depression, bipolar disorder, Tourette's syndrome, or others, you will need to have a frank discussion with her doctor about (1) additional medications for those conditions—perhaps in some cases supplanting ADHD medications; and (2) additional psychotherapies. It could be that successful treatment of her ADHD can reduce depression, but it could also be the case that her depression is serious enough to require treatment in its own right.

Heading Off Later Problems Linked with ADHD

Obviously, it's important to address the problems your preschool- or elementary-school-age daughter is experiencing right now, at this stage of life, for all the reasons discussed so far. But if we look farther ahead, we know that girls with ADHD are vulnerable to some serious problems as teenagers and adults. So it's important to target the factors that we know predict such problems while your daughter is still young. The following suggestions are based on both general findings from long-term studies of kids with ADHD and what my team and I have learned from the BGALS sample regarding female-specific factors and processes.

First, reducing ADHD symptoms is an important target. In fact, without such improvements, it may be difficult to make much headway in other domains. Both behavioral family therapy and medications can be effective in symptom reduction. Yet as emphasized throughout this book, it is especially important to help your daughter attain crucial competencies in academic performance and social skills. Simply reducing problem behaviors without active teaching and promotion of such competencies will not be sufficient, except perhaps for milder instances of ADHD in which there are no comorbid conditions present. Replacing aggressive solutions with prosocial behavior, promoting social skills, obtaining treatment to combat serious anxiety and depression (both of which erode motivation and effort), working to build reading and math skills, and promoting a less dysregulated and more supportive home environment are of the utmost importance in terms of preparing for the future.

Second, as noted in earlier chapters, one of the important negative outcomes of ADHD is an increased chance for acts of self-harm, including NSSI, through which the teenager tries to express (or mask) a deep psychological pain by injuring herself, and suicidal behavior, for which the intent is to end one's life. In a deeply distressing trend, even preteen girls are engaging in self-harm these days. Through a major substudy conducted as part of BGALS, we carefully examined the elementary-grade predictors of such outcomes:

1. The severity of both *inattentive-disorganized symptoms and hyperactive-impulsive symptoms* was implicated in risk for later self-harm—both NSSI and suicidality. Although the subgroup in BGALS with ADHD–Combined had higher risk for NSSI than the subgroup with ADHD–Inattentive, a more complete analysis revealed that the severity of inattention symptoms was also a key predictor. So, reducing such core ADHD symptoms through (for example) medication could be protective, but it's unlikely to be a complete solution. Medication effects on behavior are typically short-lived (lasting only as long as the medication is in the girl's body and brain)—and medication alone cannot promote skill building. At the same time, keeping in check the consequences of ultrasevere inattention and hyperactivity-impulsivity is a worthwhile objective.

2. *Low self-esteem* was another risk factor, regarding both NSSI and suicidal behavior. Please note that it's not worthwhile to falsely boost self-esteem

in girls (or boys) by simply telling them that they're valued and providing relatively meaningless "participation trophies." Indeed, it takes skill development and gradually increasing successes to yield real changes in one's sense of self-worth. For your daughter, doing so in a climate of encouragement, accepting and even valuing some of her differences, and building in supports outside the home are all part of the development of a more positive self-image.

3. Intriguingly, a girl's perception of the *negativity and hostility of her interactions with her dad* turned out to be another predictor of self-harmful behaviors, particularly NSSI. Of course, reducing stress and strain with either or both parents is a crucial target, but this finding highlights that supportive father–daughter interchanges are more important than one might initially think. I believe, for example, that a strong father–daughter bond can also help a vulnerable preteen girl eventually resist advances from predatory boys and help her derail early opportunities for substance use.

4. *Poor executive functions*—especially planning and problem-solving skills—predicted subsequent self-harm (again, particularly NSSI). Chapter 7 discussed means of building executive functions during school, which are important target areas.

5. *Acting out and aggressive behavior* patterns (sometimes called *externalizing behaviors*) were predictive of NSSI in later years. Finding ways of transforming negative, disruptive, and aggressive behavior patterns into prosocial actions is of the essence.

6. *Adverse experiences, particularly maltreatment,* were especially strong risk factors for later self-harm, both NSSI and suicidal behavior patterns. Doing whatever it takes to prevent physical and sexual abuse and protecting against emotional and physical neglect are of utmost importance. Other adverse experiences (separation/divorce, exposure to alcoholism, domestic violence, incarcerated parent, serious family mental illness) may not be preventable in a given household, but strong support for the girl in question is crucial.

You may remember having read about some of these risks in earlier chapters (for example, Chapter 3). But I cannot emphasize enough how beneficial it can be to engage your daughter in evidence-based treatments, as she matures, to reduce risk factors for these severe problems while you can. Your daughter's chances of thriving throughout her life could very well depend on it.

NINE

Helping Your Teenage Daughter with ADHD Thrive

This chapter focuses on girls with ADHD who are in middle school or high school, encompassing preteens and teens. Now that the often dreaded but highly important adolescent years are upon you, what will it take to promote thriving?

As noted in Chapter 3, adolescence is a time of paradox. By mid-adolescence, youth are cognitively sharper and physically more robust than they will be for the rest of their lives. The explosion of knowledge about the world, and about themselves, that emerges during this time period is staggering. Youth are literally preparing for adulthood, physically, cognitively, and emotionally. Yet adolescence is also a time of high vulnerability to impulsive actions, risky behavior, striving for independence while full self-regulation is still developing, and activities that are greatly harmful to physical and emotional maturation (substance use, risky sexual behavior, self-harm, accidental injury, and the like).

As I highlighted early in this book, it is now clearly known that ADHD does not end with puberty. Although your daughter's physical activity levels may decline, ongoing disorganization, forgetfulness, and impulse-control issues can not only perpetuate existing problems but add new ones. In fact, impairments often mount during adolescence, when high school presents huge demands for organization and independence, even though symptoms may seem to taper off, especially in the area of motor movement. Talk about a "mixed" time of life!

All this is a good reason to embrace the perspective that ADHD is not just a group of inattentive and hyperactive-impulsive symptoms but a fundamental issue of self-control that can make life adjustment difficult as expectations for independence and for close relationships increase during the teen years. To make things even tougher for your teenage daughter, coordinating the behavioral treatment that is often so helpful among multiple classrooms and teachers, along with a host of after-school activities, can be a heavy lift.

> *Your daughter's self-control problems may intensify during adolescence—just when it becomes more complicated to provide the behavioral therapy that can help.*

Chapter 3 highlighted the pernicious "triple bind" that snares so many preadolescent and adolescent girls, who face competing (and unsolvable) demands for being (1) nurturing, (2) super-competitive, and (3) relentlessly effortless and sexualized while trying to do both. The costs—in terms of lowered self-esteem, internalization of failure, and sheer exhaustion—are often considerable. The triple bind is even more difficult to negotiate for a girl lacking in fundamental aspects of self-regulation, whose psychological and behavioral development lags behind her physical development and actual age.

The Demands of Adolescence

Adolescence imposes a host of demands (and conflicts) on all developing girls, but they can be particularly tough for a daughter who is showing the signs of (or has been diagnosed with) ADHD:

- *Organization:* The name of the game in middle school and high school is, quite simply: Get organized . . . and stay organized! This is a major challenge for all youth. Yet for those with ADHD—who struggle to remember assignments, who misplace things constantly, who never seem to have a semblance of an organized binder, and whose teachers frequently remark that "she's smart enough, but she just can't get the message as to what the assignments really are"—organization and time management are key challenges. At the same time, it's far harder to get five or six different teachers, each teaching a different subject, on board with organizational supports for your daughter with ADHD than it was with a single grade-school teacher each year.

- *Academic demands:* As you may recall from your own experiences in secondary school, academic subjects become far more difficult and challenging. History and its interlocking themes; algebra, geometry, trig (and beyond); grammar and literary devices; current biology, chemistry, and physics; advanced foreign languages; and the many electives (and AP classes) of high school are among the mix. If your daughter is not attending to the material, remembering and sequencing her assignments, taking good notes in key classes, staying ahead of the game via homework, and planning for term-long projects, she'll soon be struggling just to tread water.

• *Friendships and intimate relationships:* Your daughter is now likely to be engaged in a relatively large school setting with far more peers than ever before. As puberty hits, desires for contact—emotional and physical—flare. How to negotiate this new biological reality and the new partner-related terrain it encompasses is a major task for everyone. But girls who have been ostracized by peers from grade school onward (or girls with the primarily inattentive form of ADHD, who simply may not be as engaged or connected with peers) could be lacking practice in developing social skills. Reading social cues, dealing with rejection (and the likelihood of relational aggression—teasing, reputation damaging, being excluded), and handling pressure for sexual behavior are all huge hurdles. Because of the inherent value that most girls place on social connectedness, failures and rejection in this domain can take a huge toll on your daughter's self-concept and self-esteem.

• *The world of social media:* Most parents (including me!) have little if any true idea of the warp-speed-paced, click-and-swipe, and volatile nature of the many forms of social media that teens now encounter each hour (make that each minute) of the day. Research shows that if a teen has close in-person relationships, social media can enhance the value of such contacts. But if the primary means of relating to peers is online, loneliness and potential isolation are likely with increasing reliance on virtual contacts. In fact, some of the best research on this topic—though now several years old—is that girls with ADHD "overuse" social media compared to their peers. More recent data reveal that Instagram use, in particular, can fuel mental health problems in teen girls because of the social comparisons that tend to get made with respect to the "perfect" images encountered (see *https://theguardian.com/technology/2021/sep/18/ teenage-girls-body-image-and-instagrams-perfect-storm*). Such use can promote the sense that one isn't living up to the images constantly seen online regarding the looks, popularity, and "social capital" of others who seem to be making it all work—reminiscent of the triple bind (see Chapter 3). Finally, social media can make permanent any record of a misstep, potentially fueling rumination about it, which can fuel depression and low self-worth in girls.

• *Sleep deprivation:* At present, academic standards are raised ever higher (check out the ridiculously low rates of college admissions to elite schools these days), along with mounting pressures, constant multitasking, and multiple extracurricular activities (including athletics). So, it's little wonder that a frank majority of teens (both girls and boys) get nowhere near the nine hours of sleep per night recommended during adolescence. Moreover, ADHD itself can contribute to sleep difficulties. The combination can be devastating. Indeed, research reveals that sleep deprivation is a core trigger for experiencing and expressing negative emotions over and above positive emotions—and for decreases in memory functions.

• *Family stress and strife:* Evolution predicts that teens crave independence. Over the last century, the average age at which girls reach puberty has decreased by two years or so, but at the same time, today's world demands longer periods of education, paired with delays in careers and childbearing. So, what's left is a huge gap—that is, earlier physical maturation paired with an ever-increasing span of time prior to psychosocial and economic independence. As a result, family life can be extremely stressful when a teen is in the picture. And if your daughter has the kinds of self-regulatory deficits that are the hallmark of ADHD, family stress may well magnify during adolescence. As well, core issues of curfews; sexual experimentation; the ready presence of nicotine, alcohol, weed (marijuana), and harder drugs; and choice of peer group members are a major part of the landscape, too often compounding family stress to the max.

• *Driving:* Although some research reveals that teenage girls with ADHD may not share the same driving-related risks as do teenage boys with ADHD, there's still plenty of reason for concern. In short, is it worth having a 16-year-old girl, whose executive functions and brain development may well lag behind those of her peers by several years, managing a several-thousand-pound motor vehicle on crowded streets? And make sure not to respond to the latest text message while doing so? There's not space here to engage in any kind of debate about what the legal driving age should be, or whether youth with impairments in focus, judgment, and impulse control

> *Teen girls with ADHD are striving for independence just like other girls—but their ability to handle independence may lag several years behind that of other girls their age.*

should have to wait longer than others to attain this privilege. Still, you may want to consider the contingencies you would have in place for your daughter to get a learner's permit and then license (for example, if she takes ADHD medication successfully, will she be able to drive only while taking it?).

The teen years are indeed a time of major challenges. So much so that parents of a teenage girl with ADHD sometimes find themselves slipping into a pattern of harsh communication and judgment about their child (especially true for parents of a girl with the combined presentation of ADHD, but certainly possible with respect to the inattentive presentation, too). This is not a reflection of lack of love for your daughter. Rather, it is a product of unresolved stress on the family. Expressing anger and frustration is rarely intentional on the parents' part. But that does not mean it should be allowed to continue.

At All Costs, Don't Invalidate Your Daughter

When things get rough at home with a girl who is impulsive and defiant, or even a girl who is passive and noncompliant, parental expectations for having a responsive, "normal" daughter usually get lowered. And the perception, too often, is that the daughter "has it in" for the parent.

- She *must* be able to act more reasonably!
- She *can't* disobey or fail to listen unless she's trying to do me in.
- Something's *fundamentally wrong* with her. Or with me and our whole family.

These feelings and attributions can lead some parents into *harshly criticizing* their daughter and even *invalidating* her perspectives on herself and life.

For example:

- "You've had it in for me since you were little. What on earth is the matter with you?"
- "You've never appreciated, for even one moment, all that we've done for you."
- In the aftermath of a harsh punishment: "That's not the way it happened—I never got that angry with you, I was just trying to teach

you some lessons." Or "You deserved it and you know it. No child in our family would ever think that we would be cruel to you."

When statements like this begin to take over parent–daughter interactions (or parent–son interactions), the preteen or teen may come to doubt her own sense of reality and identity. She may also come to believe that she's so inherently bad that her own parent doesn't really see that she has independent views and feelings. Especially if she has ADHD, she may come to blame herself intensely, even though she doesn't yet have the full insight as to her own lapses in self-regulation.

Crucially, such invalidating and harshly critical parent–child interactions are involved in pathways to both self-injurious behavior (that is, NSSI and suicidal behavior patterns) and externalizing, acting-out behavior. They are not the only causal factor, of course, but they can play an insidious and important role.

How to avoid this outcome? As difficult as it may seem, try the following.

- Pause before making an "escalating," defensive, angry response. Ask yourself: "What is it that I really want to communicate?"
- Rehearse what you really want to say. For example, it's OK to say you're angry, and it's OK to recognize that your daughter may be angry with a limit you set—but don't meet fire with fire.
- Try to de-escalate.
- Pose curious, genuine questions about her behavior patterns. And listen to her answers.
- Look for positives and small signs of progress in communication.
- Believe in your daughter's integrity.
- Try to see your daughter for who she is.

Taking the last measure may involve a kind of *radical acceptance* that your daughter has some core differences from most other girls, a topic raised in Chapter 1. In fact, it may take considerable collaboration plus real effort on your part to show warmth and limits, in order to turn things around. In short, it's *radical acceptance* paired with *radical commitment* on your part.

Overall, during heated moments, try to work on turning the temperature way down and reconstructing a set of positive expectations, narratives, and contingencies in your home. All this doesn't mean that you back down but instead that you listen, reply in a responsive manner, and work toward gradual change, without a yelling and screaming match and without devaluing or invalidating your daughter.

> As pressures on her to achieve multiply, it's more important than ever for your daughter to feel valued by you.

Maddie (age 14 and diagnosed with ADHD–Combined since age 7) and her mom are going at it verbally. The (yelled) topics include Maddie's abandoning ninth-grade schoolwork, violating house rules, staying out late, and seeing several classmates for "dates." Family stress and strain, and lots of mutual denigration, are on full display.

Interaction Style to Avoid

Mom: *Maddie, it's 11:00 on a Tuesday night. Where have you been? What the hell are you doing with your life?* (escalating to a scream) *Just what is going on with you? I don't see my daughter anymore—just a profane, defiant girl who looks like my daughter. Do I really know you?*

Maddie: *Oh yeah, then why did you even have a daughter? All you want to do is control me.*

Mom: *I want a daughter who's a human being, not someone I don't even know. How can you even be in our family if these people you're seeing are doing drugs and watching porn? Who are you?*

Clearly, this pattern reflects mutual escalation. No one will win, and both mom and daughter will end up defeated and full of self-blame.

Interaction Styles to Try Out Instead

Mom: *Wait, let's slow down. You know that our home contract says that you have to be home by 9:30 on school nights. [More on home contracts later in this chapter.] This is the second time this week you've been late. I need to have your iPhone, now. It's in the contract.*

Maddie: *WHAT? Mom, I NEED my phone! My school assignments are on it!*

Mom: *Here's the contract—look here. I will take it for 24 hours, and you can get your assignments on your laptop.*

Maddie: *Damn you, Mom, you just don't get it. I didn't grow up in the Dark Ages like you.*

Mom: (ignoring Maddie's swearing at her) *Maddie, you know how much I love you. But I want you to be safe, and this is what we agreed on.*

Maddie: *I'm my own boss.*

Mom: *Maybe that's your view, but as long as you live here, we have certain rules.*

Maddie: *Hey, Mom, you're so old that you don't even think that a ninth-grader can watch porn.*

Mom: (trying to be reflective rather than reactive) *Hold on. I'm interested. What did you watch? What was it like?*

Moral: Be firm but also be curious. Responding with harsh judgment to a difficult topic, or one around which shame is often present, will send a clear signal to your daughter never to speak with you about that topic again. Over the next moments, Maddie sensed that her mom was actually interested in her experiences and slowed down at times to talk with her. All this led to a more mature set of conversations between Mom and Maddie about her home contract, her desire for independence, her sexuality, and her love/hate relationship with her family's limits.

When any teen, and especially one with ADHD, sees that her parents are genuinely interested in her—and therefore doesn't have to prove her independence by defying any parental rules—a different home environment can emerge. All this takes work, patience, practice, and realizing how important it is to blend warmth with limits.

Preventive "Medicine": Focus on Strengths

When your developing daughter is a preteen, keep in mind that the increasing independence of mind and behavior that signals adolescence can also be strengths for girls with ADHD *if clear supports and structure are in place—and if she has good outlets for what she's really good at.*

Above all, I cannot emphasize the following strongly enough: **Spending time with your teenage daughter to discuss and identify strengths— including high-interest activities, favored school subjects, hobbies, and extracurriculars in which she thrives—is time *extremely* well spent.** Too often, the main focus is on problems. But when your daughter is engaged in such positive actions, she will be highly likely to get naturally rewarded for her strong efforts toward that subject or activity. Such intrinsic motivation can help her develop a greater sense of confidence and competence.

In other words, helping your teenage daughter thrive is not just about remediating areas of weakness. Also essential is building on strengths and interests and finding the best environments in which your daughter "fits," both of which can help right now and even in planning future endeavors for her. You will undoubtedly also find that focusing on what your daughter does well, and enjoys, is an antidote to any tendency to shift toward the negative in your interactions with her.

> *Look for your daughter's strengths, providing as many opportunities as possible to build on them.*

Much of the rest of this chapter deals with the kinds of interventions that can help with problem behavior and promote thriving. Yet psychologists and other mental health professionals like me often spend too much time on treating problems and not enough time on enhancing skills and strengths. Remember to look for and promote areas of strength!

Digging Up Hidden Interests

The downward spiral for Kay had been building for some years. Shy and a bit socially awkward beginning in preschool, she was an only child who had never been able to follow multipart directions well at home and often appeared isolated in the neighborhood where other girls gathered to play. She received a truly mixed bag of teacher evaluations in kindergarten and elementary school, most of which carried the underlying message that if she could only tune in—and focus—she would show a whole lot more learning. And, other teachers said, ... her desk is completely cluttered . . . it's a miracle she can find anything . . . if only she could become more organized.

During grade school, she barely completed her homework, woke up later than she should (enduring her mom's pleas to get in the car on time for school), and seemed even lonelier. Once, at the end of fourth grade, her mom overheard Kay saying to a classmate on her cell phone—should fourth graders even have cell phones? her mom wondered—that she sometimes thought she'd be better off if she weren't alive, because no one liked her. Her mom barged in, and Kay bashfully said that she didn't really mean it—she just wondered why she always messed everything up. Even so, her mother was concerned.

Not long afterward, and coincidentally, a family friend, whose daughter just happened to be a classmate of Kay's, made a class observation/visit. On the phone that evening with Kay's mom, she remarked that Kay reminded her of her own niece, a sweet girl who seemed lost in class and unsure of herself in peer groups. She went on to say that her niece had been diagnosed with the inattentive presentation of ADHD in seventh grade—and that although the accommodations (including expectations for shorter bursts of homework each evening) had been helpful, the family wished that they had known about these issues when she was still in elementary school.

Kay's mom, a single parent, looked up local support groups for ADHD and began to learn that, in many girls, ADHD doesn't really fit the "boy" stereotype of rambunctious, defiant behavior patterns. A local pediatrician, with specialty training in developmental/behavioral pediatrics, performed a careful evaluation and said that Kay clearly met criteria for ADHD–Inattentive, with a building set of symptoms nearing the range of major depression as well.

The treatment plan included a course of behavioral family therapy, support for Kay's apparent depression, and a wait-and-see-until approach until the fall of fifth grade for a decision on medication. By mid-fall, with grades no better—and with Kay's mom frustrated that the reward charts didn't seem to be taking hold—the doctor prescribed a low dosage of a nonstimulant medication, guanfacine. It was hard to see any clearly positive results. Later in the school year, the doctor took her off that medication and began a trial of a low dose of stimulant. Through twice-weekly teacher ratings, some small improvements in attention and direction-following were apparent.

Yet sixth grade and middle school uncovered additional problems. Kay had seemingly no idea how to shift from her "core" English/history teacher in the morning to her math/science teacher in the afternoon. The larger class sizes, and the physically bigger and more mature fellow sixth-grade classmates, made Kay feel even lonelier and more withdrawn.

Another chance occurrence: In mid-fall, Kay was asked by the parent of a preschool acquaintance of Kay's, named Andrea—who had now rejoined her at the large new middle school—to come along on a Saturday afternoon trip to a horse farm. Although initially reticent, saying that she hadn't seen Andrea since she was 5 years old and that Andrea hadn't really reached out to her in middle school, Kay reluctantly agreed.

That evening, Kay's mother had never seen Kay so animated. Kay went on and on about the wonderful horses and other animals around the farm, talking about how one of the farmhands let her help wash and groom a beautiful mare. Kay's mom had never dared to get Kay a pet, fearing that Kay might inadvertently neglect it. But now, quickly putting two and two together, she started to ask Kay about other experiences with animals at friends' homes or during outings. Each time Kay glowed.

As a reward on her DRC for middle school, Kay's mom decided to add a new incentive: With a consistent majority of yes responses over the next two weeks, Kay could earn a trip to a local pet store. After that success, which eventually ended with a pet dog, the next incentive was a repeat trip to the horse farm. This was another "large" reward, and Kay's efforts required several weeks of hard work. Her mom recalled what seemed to have been empty words of the behavioral therapist the previous year: "Once your kid has a reward she really desires, she will show strong effort."

Even more, although never an avid reader, Kay and her mom met with the core English/history teacher, who helped Kay find books on animals throughout history, as well as basic animal husbandry, which Kay actually asked to read at night, past her usual bedtime. The teacher also suggested some other girls at school, in sixth and seventh grade, with similar interests, as potential connections for Kay. Amazingly, to her mom, Kay's motivation began to soar. And Kay and Andrea began to be friends.

Have her ADHD issues and problems vanished? No, of course not, but this newfound interest and purpose have started to pull Kay out of her shell and get her engaged in learning. Back at the horse farm, she's begun to inquire about what age she must be to begin some part-time work. Maybe, her mom now thinks, there's more hope for Kay's future.

Of course, not everyone has a "retreat" at a horse farm. For other girls, it might be engagement in drama activities—and working with a younger brother or younger kids at school to get them involved. Alternatively, maybe sports—or cooking—is the true "outlet." Anything you can do to foster opportunities and engagement can go a long way toward helping your daughter develop important lifelong interests and a sense of intrinsic motivation for something at which she thrives. Such activities (as was horse grooming for Kay) can also serve as powerful rewards for her home program/contract.

Behavioral Family Therapy with Teens

The family supports required for teenage girls with ADHD need to be more flexible and negotiation-heavy during the teen years than those in place with the "refrigerator charts" that provided assistance during elementary school. As ADHD-in-teens expert Maggie Sibley contends, the optimal stance is one of collaboration with your daughter rather than (1) overcontrolling her, (2) doing too much for her, or (3) essentially letting her go without any supports at all. During the adolescent period, adult involvement is still crucial for intervention with teenage ADHD, but it should include a gradual handoff of responsibilities to the adolescent, as she works toward growing autonomy.

Work with teens displaying ADHD is all about negotiation, showing warmth and support, promoting strengths, setting mutual goals, collaborative efforts, clear limits and enforcing them . . . and then more negotiation. At the same time, it's also crucial not to get impatient or frustrated when progress is slow or erratic, which can lead to giving up at the first signs of setback. As shown in Maddie's story (see pages 210–211), it's about setting up contracts with desired rewards, too. You're playing a long game here, in a period of huge transition for your daughter and the entire family.

I should add that many parents get wary, as their daughter gets older, of angering or provoking her by setting any limits at all. But please recall the principles underlying authoritative parenting (see Chapter 5), through which warmth and responsiveness are buttressed and balanced by appropriate controls and limit setting. The ways in which you show warmth may well shift over time (perhaps fewer long hugs but a greater number of more supportive, specific comments). Similarly, limits are likely to be far different from the physical restraining from danger for a preschooler who bolts toward the street or the points subtracted from a reward chart or DRC back in third grade. Such limits include clear messages in the contract you negotiate with your daughter (see below) regarding the consequences for her failing to live up to her end of the expectations. Adolescent behavior management requires a gradual relinquishing of the kinds of controls needed for a younger girl, while still maintaining appropriate monitoring of her whereabouts and having clear consequences in your contract with her when she violates its terms. Again, behavior management at this age requires rewards that carry real impact.

During the adolescent years, teens need to be granted more autonomy as they progress to adulthood. Additionally, the large numbers of teachers in the lives of most middle-school and high-school students make coordinated home–school efforts difficult. Furthermore, although keeping tabs on your daughter is crucial, no parent can monitor their teenage daughter 24/7 (much as some parents might like to). For all of these reasons, behavioral family therapy programs not only require modification for teens, but usually need to be supplemented by additional, adolescent-specific programs—some of which, importantly, encourage parental involvement as well (see the section "Adolescent-Focused Programs" on page 224).

In the transition from childhood to adolescence, crucial issues regarding behavioral family treatment and other specific treatments for girls with ADHD include the following.

● Begin to replace the refrigerator charts with *contracts*—in which parents clarify their requirements for thriving at home, while the daughter makes clear what she expects to get in return. A contract is a kind of "family legal document" as opposed to a parent-led reward chart. Give-and-take is of the essence. What I mean here is that just as you, as the parent, write in the contract your expectations for home rules, learning, and thriving, your daughter in turn lists what she expects from you in terms of growing independence and rewards for meeting your goals (please see "Negotiating a Contract," pages 218–221, for a concrete example).

● Contracts require sensitive negotiation with your daughter: What are the core responsibilities and chores you expect her to complete? What are the critical academic standards to uphold in the home? What are the limits with respect to being home at certain times as adolescence progresses? In parallel, what are the expectations that your daughter desires from *you*—in terms of not invading her privacy? Or figuring out the right amount of allowance money? Or gaining your gradual trust related to her wish for growing independence?

● In this process, remember that your daughter may still be several years behind her peers in terms of self-regulation, intrinsic motivation, organizational skills, and restraint over her impulses for independence. Your ultimate aim is, of course, to prepare her for a more independent life ahead, but in the meantime, you may need to deal with resistance on her part related to *any* reasonable controls and limits you impose.

● Behavioral family therapy cannot do all of the skill teaching and performance coaching that teens require. In fact, there are a growing number of evidence-based treatments for teens with ADHD, focusing on maladaptive thinking strategies, bolstering organizational skills, improving social communication, and more (see next section). There's a lot you can do at home, but school supports and community-level programs are also a key part of the mix.

> *Adolescence is the time to shift from parent-led reward charts to mutually negotiated contracts, as you gradually relinquish some control to your daughter.*

Staying engaged with your daughter is of the essence. Many experts in behavioral family therapy for adolescents with ADHD call for the youth to attend, if not all, at least a number of therapist–parent sessions, to promote their more active engagement. In some forms of CBT, for example, a key goal is to help parents better understand their teen's attitudes and "headsets" about ADHD and the world—and on the flip side, to help teens understand why their parents are still so "concerned" and "demanding" and "unfair."

Preteen girls with ADHD entering middle school may still do well with the kinds of reward programs you instituted when they were in grade school. Included here are DRCs. Soon enough, though, your daughter's burgeoning sense of independence may prompt her to recoil from being treated like a child. She will wish to participate, as a near-equal partner, in negotiating (1) your goals for greater organization, independence, and academic performance alongside (2) her goals for the kinds of respect and rewards she will earn for progress in these domains. Again, a contract is a mutual document in which you outline your expectations for better performance and behavioral control—with, once again, reasonable steps for success, especially at the beginning—and she in turn writes down what she expects to earn for meeting such expectations.

Find neutral times, devoid of anger and blaming (on both your side and her side), during which you sit down and draft both your expectations and your daughter's, along with the expected rewards once she meets her goals. If you're still working with a behavioral family therapist, engage this therapist deeply in the process.

Because you're the parent, you may want your daughter to become totally in love with the middle-school or high-school classes in which she's enrolled, working diligently without any external contingencies or rewards. But, of course, no teen is enamored of all of her classes. And if your daughter has ADHD, which may involve delays in brain development, maturation, and intrinsic motivation that can last far beyond childhood, interest may lag even more. So, on the parental side, a contract requires the same kind of gradually increasing goals and expectations—as I've said throughout, Rome was not built in a day—that can lead to gradual longer-term gains. On the teen's side, the contract requires extrinsic motivators (rewards) that other girls her age may no longer need but that are still necessary for her development of self-regulation. She will also want you to respect her growing independence.

Negotiating a Contract

Letitia is a tenth-grade girl, formally diagnosed with ADHD in seventh grade. Looking back, her parents have come to wonder how she made it through grade school without getting a diagnosis. Every year her teacher would talk about her spark and potential, along with "pushing the limits," but her academic grades ranged from A to D, once she started getting actual letter grades in third grade. Even her first- and second-grade report cards ranged from ecstasy with respect to certain parts of the curriculum to near agony for others. Struggles in math were present each year. She was finally diagnosed with ADHD–Combined, because of both serious inattention and plenty of impulsive behavior, along with a possible learning disorder in math, plus anxious and oppositional "tendencies."

In retrospect, once Letitia was in middle school, the single teacher her school district offered for sixth-graders had barely kept her afloat. With multiple teachers per day after that, all bets were off.

Work with a behavioral therapist in seventh and eighth grades, who led both individual and group sessions, helped the family establish a DRC and a 504 plan. Letitia also received a relatively low dose of Concerta during those years, which helped with her organization and facilitated a more compliant attitude toward home-based rules. It also helped her focus better in algebra and geometry classes at school, though she continued to struggle in both.

Ninth grade marked the transition to a large urban high school. She did better than expected during her initial semester, but sophomore and junior boys started noticing her, and some of her fellow girls started calling her "weird" when she confessed that she was taking medication for ADHD. She had a habit of yelling back at any teacher who corrected her in class. One of her female friends let her know that weed is better for focusing on homework and "chilling" from anxiety than any medicines prescribed by a doctor. To her parents' great consternation, Letitia began to refuse taking her morning Concerta. She also started smoking weed during occasional weekend parties.

By March of tenth grade, Letitia's parents noticed a drop-off in motivation for schoolwork and homework, along with increased hostility toward any requests they made at home. Grades had been in decline since the end of the first semester. With their concern rising, they recontacted their behavioral therapist, who had expertise in working with teens. Letitia reluctantly agreed to attend a couple of family sessions. The focus was on forging a home contract.

The therapist worked hard with Letitia and her parents to find a few initial target behaviors rather than attempt to take on the deluge of rising issues all at once. Here's some sample dialogue from the therapy sessions:

Mom: *Letitia, we just don't know what's come over you since the fall. You used to care more about yourself and get help for your ADHD. But we don't know where you are these days.*

Letitia: *Geez, Mom, lay off. Can't you understand that all my friends are sick of their parents' freaking out about them? So what if guys might be into me? So what if I don't meet your expectations to get all A's?*

Therapist: *I'm hearing that your mom is concerned, Letitia. Mom, can you speak to the feeling behind that?*

Mom: *I love you, Letitia, but you're pulling away from us so fast. Don't you see that we're just trying to help?*

Dad: *I love you, too, Letitia, but the arguing at home is just making me want to spend more and more time at work. Not that the family doesn't need more income these days.*

Therapist: *Letitia, can you hear the caring and love in your parents' statements?*

Letitia: *I guess so, but it just feels like everyone is hassling me. I need some space.*

The behavioral therapist reflects on both the parental concern and love and Letitia's desire for greater independence. She then begins modeling how a contract is made, different from Letitia's middle-school reward chart (even though based on similar principles). Through patient work, she helps Letitia see that the parents actually do want the best for her—and helps the parents realize that Letitia is not still a preteen.

Therapist: *OK, Letitia, what are the things that you most want from your family right now?*

Letitia: *For them to let me be my own person.*

Therapist: *Let's get more specific. How could they show that?*

Letitia: *By not barging into my room to inspect that it's spotless all the time. I mean, come on!*

Therapist: *Anything else?*

Letitia: *Yeah, could they stop criticizing me all day and night?*

Therapist: *Let's write these out on the contract.*

More specific actions are added to the contract, as the therapist asks Letitia to dictate these expectations in her own words.

Therapist (after typing out Letitia's requests): *OK, Mom and Dad, do these seem like reasonable requests that you can address?* (acknowledging the parents' nods, she goes on) *And what are two starting points for you, in terms of Letitia?*

Dad: *Well, we would want her to show us her completed homework at night, before we start arguing with her, and if it's done, we add a check on her reward chart. Can we make that part of the contract?*

Mom: *I agree. Maybe we can get updates from each teacher as to last night's homework, so we don't have to keep bugging you, Letitia.*

Therapist: *And what if you can show your parents the completed homework, Letitia? What reward would you want?*

The conversation continues as the family negotiates a reward of extra allowance, and extra time at friends' on weekends, if Letitia is up to date on homework completion.

Therapist: *Another goal, Mom and Dad?*

Mom: *Well, Letitia, I've noticed that you just don't want to take your ADHD medication any longer. Why not?*

At this point, given the openness and trust that have begun to emerge from the negotiation, Letitia backs down somewhat from her previous stance that the Concerta is stifling her creativity and says the following:

Letitia: *You know, I actually liked getting better grades. I also looked at some of the YouTubes from Simone Biles about her ADHD. Maybe I should try those pills again.*

Mom: *If you did, maybe we'd all learn whether they still make a difference for your focusing. Would you be willing to talk with your doctor about it?*

Letitia: *OK, maybe—when's my next appointment?*

The therapist comments on the give-and-take during this revealing interaction, adding to the contract that if Letitia agrees to restart the medication on a trial basis, the family will be open to adding an extended time, this coming summer, to a vacation on which a friend's family has invited Letitia.

Note that I've condensed the time frame above. Many such negotiations take more time and patience than the scenario just presented. But the core principles are clear: Treat your teenage daughter with respect and independence and set out reasonable and attainable goals as you embark on the contract. Make sure that you maintain your "end" of the contract's bargaining points, too, by working to respect her independence in the ways laid out in your negotiations. The reward chart may need to be more subtle than the ones that used to decorate the refrigerator in the kitchen. Do not "cave" on your basic expectations. And listen carefully for your daughter's side of the negotiations as you strive to come up with a plan that's workable for all.

Above all, show your love and respect for your daughter, even if such love has been challenged by trying times and a trying history. The only way to go is forward.

Note: If there are added comorbid conditions (for example, if Letitia is also experiencing serious depression, or if she is engaging in self-harming behaviors), then additional interventions—such as CBT for depression, DBT, medications beyond ADHD meds—may well need to be tried. One of the difficult clinical questions in working with teens with ADHD (or people with ADHD of any age, for that matter) is where to put primary focus: on the ADHD-related issues or on the comorbid condition(s) that also exist? There's no hard-and-fast answer, but the set of problems requiring the most attention and yielding the greatest impairment may need to be tackled first.

Avoiding Coercion

There is a particularly difficult pattern of parent–child interaction that can develop when increasingly aggressive behaviors occur in a preteen or teenage girl with ADHD. Typically, such parent–child interactions show up in a girl (or boy) who is quite oppositional from an early age (a kid more likely to have ADHD–Combined than ADHD–Inattentive). The underlying point is that parents start tiptoeing around limit setting through ineffective bouts of reminding, nagging, and the like. The underlying reason is that they may fear an explosive reaction if they set really firm limits. The daughter views these half-hearted attempts to control her as annoying and frustrating—finally escalating to a threat of violence, or of leaving the home, which serves to get the parents to back off from their (largely ineffective) demands. This pattern has been called *coercion,* and it's truly a vicious cycle.

Preventing Coercion by Staying True to Your Limits

Alison showed real signs of ADHD, as well as oppositional behavior, at age 4. Frankly, she hasn't really let up over the years (she's now 16). That is, the tantrums and refusals at preschool, the suspensions in elementary school for serious rule violations, and detours into intensive weed smoking and alcohol use in middle school have now morphed into hanging with the wrong crowd as a high-school sophomore, with a juvenile record for violations of curfew and stealing beers from neighbors and local stores.

Her single-parent dad had the sense, when he and his now-deceased wife adopted her at age 2 (following several foster placements), that Alison would never be an easy child. The records back then, as limited as they were, revealed a teenage biological mom (with a history of ADHD and substance abuse herself), early neglect, and no secure early attachments. Alison's inability to focus and her utter lack of impulse control were consistent with ADHD, along with the effects of trauma.

A typical interaction at home:

Dad: *Alison, please at least try to do your homework! You barely passed ninth grade—do you want to fail sophomore year?*

Alison: *Damn it, Dad, mellow out! I hate school. I have enough bad stuff going on in my life.*

Dad: *Come on, be reasonable. And don't talk with me that way.*

Alison: *I'll talk with you any way I want unless you back off.*

Dad has not enforced the contract-based limit of Alison losing her cell phone for a day if homework isn't done in a clear time frame—and he's increasingly terrified of her reactions. He might actually lose his daughter if she's pushed too far, fearing that she could run out and he'd never see her again. Maybe he'd lose real contact with her forever. So he continues to soft-pedal.

Dad: *Let's start again. Don't you want to graduate from high school?*

Alison: *Maybe, but I won't if you keep pestering me.*

Dad's beginning to boil over:

Dad: (starting to yell) *Alison, I have just had it. Do your homework or else!*

Alison: (clearly egging him on) *Or else what?*

Dad: *I'll kick you out or smack some sense into you!*

Alison: *Oh yeah? I dare you!*

At that, Dad lashes out to slap her on the face. She recoils, avoiding most of the blow, then storms out of the house, saying "Don't try to find me—I'm never coming back."

Over the years, Dad has cared deeply for Alison yet has been worried, even terrified about her future. He clearly realized from parent support meetings back when she was much younger that she had a genetic risk for ADHD compounded by huge early trauma. But especially after his wife, Alison's adoptive mother, died of cancer when Alison was in second grade, he has been increasingly afraid of triggering her. Although he went to behavior management classes, he could never seem to hold to a limit, fearful of her explosive reaction.

In this pattern of coercive interaction, a child (and later a teen) with ADHD—who typically experiences lots of externalizing (aggressive) problems as well—manages to get away with noncompliant behavior because of ineffective limits and consequences. Finally, when she pushes back so hard that the parent loses control, a rupture occurs. Alison obviously needs trauma-informed therapy and the medication that she always refused to take. At the same time, the coercion just depicted fuels her externalizing behavior—and may well engender self-harming tendencies.

All this emphasizes the importance of childhood and early-adolescent intervention to increase warmth and validation, while simultaneously delivering real consequences when the behavior has not met the home standard.

Adolescent-Focused Programs

By the mid- to late teen years, your daughter may be ready to go beyond some of the externally driven, parent- and teacher-led, reward-based behavioral programs that marked her childhood. For example, she can engage in CBT, which will help her to take active ownership of work on organizational skills and time management, to work on replacing negative and self-defeating thoughts with positive ones, and to engage in strategies related to anger management and other forms of self-control as needed. There are also additional adolescent-based programs that can be of real benefit. Some of these are for "consumption" by adolescents with ADHD themselves; others engage parents, to ensure some consistency across a girl's life. In fact, just because one or more of the teen-specific treatments is available to your daughter does *not* mean that you as a parent should disengage. On the contrary, though she may not voice it directly (and may in fact appear to be doing her best to distance from you), she actually needs you and your authoritative guidance—and appropriate monitoring—more than ever during her teen years.

> Your daughter may benefit from programs designed specifically for teens, but that doesn't mean she no longer needs your support and your willingness to listen.

Your daughter also needs to know that you're there to listen to her. Sometimes, by keeping an open stance and not hounding her into disclosing all that she feels, parents can get an unexpected invitation for a conversation about hopes, fears, doubts, and more. And, as noted earlier, taking a curious stance (rather than overreacting to subjects she brings up that you find offensive) may actually encourage her to be more open with you.

CBT

Two decades ago, pioneering clinicians in Boston and New York developed and investigated the applicability of CBT to adults with ADHD. (Recall that, through the 1970s and 1980s, there was serious doubt that ADHD even persisted into adulthood—so why would anyone bother adapting CBT principles for adults with ADHD?). Within the past 10-plus years, innovations have escalated, so that "packages" of CBT have been tested with adolescents diagnosed with ADHD, whether they receive medication or not. Results are promising. A key example is the program from Massachusetts General Hospital for adults with ADHD, with subsequent modifications for teens. These procedures have been tested in an individual therapy format. Notably, parents are brought into several full sessions throughout the 12-week program—and they are also invited in at the end of every session, so that they are fully aware of the skills their teen is learning.

Modules include the following:

1. *Psychoeducation and organization/planning:* Here teens learn some of the same material on ADHD presented in early chapters of this book and are given instruction in using paper or electronic planners, in prompting and reminding themselves of portions of assignments that are due, and in planning ahead.

2. *Controlling distractibility:* Among other procedures, therapists encourage teens to choose reasonable goals for a given assignment (such as homework), use timers to guide themselves, and place cell phones and other distractions aside for the work period.

3. *Adaptive thinking:* CBT for adults involves recording helpful and unhelpful thoughts. Teens are taught to be alert for a critical "inner coach" who either promotes rumination ("Look at how you screwed that up") or instructs the teen to put off working on an assignment because there's plenty of time to finish it when, in fact, some work needs to be done each day.

4. *Stopping procrastination:* Through thought modification and realistic planning, and dealing with perfectionistic thinking, the teen works to avoid putting off work until the last minute.

Homework Interventions (and More)

Evidence-based treatments for enhancing homework skills and homework completion for teens with ADHD have shown real effectiveness. One such program is the after-school Challenging Horizons Program. This is a "homework-plus" program, primarily for middle-school students, which meets two to three afternoons per week for an entire school year. It is actually a blended program that features, beyond homework coaching, social goal setting and planning. The after-school staff provides reinforcers in the form of snacks, or participation in recreational activities, for students making progress. Another program is the Homework, Organization, and Planning Skills (HOPS) program, delivered during the school day by school psychologists/counselors, in relatively short sessions (16 of them). It is also for middle-school students, though recent modifications for high-school students with ADHD have been examined. HOPS now includes direct parental involvement, so that parents can learn to promote homework completion after the school day ends. Each program involves instruction in how to use binders, bookbags, and locker storage, with plentiful checklists and reminders and rewards for the teens who learn these skills.

Supporting Teens' Autonomy Daily

Maggie Sibley of the University of Washington created Supporting Teens' Autonomy Daily (STAND), a multiweek program explicitly targeting teens with ADHD and their parents. STAND blends the following: behavioral family therapy, a more traditional family therapy approach that emphasizes mutual communication, organizational skills training for the teen, and an important procedure called motivational interviewing (MI). MI is a strategy that goes far beyond ADHD: It involves directed questioning of family members about their own issues (and ambivalences) about making change in core life domains (for example, engaging in substance abuse). In the words of some of its developers: "It is a collaborative, goal-oriented style of communication with particular attention to the language of change. It is designed to strengthen personal motivation for and commitment to a specific goal by eliciting and exploring the person's own reasons for change within an atmosphere of acceptance and compassion" (Miller & Rollnick, 2013, p. 29).

In other words, rather than suggest or cajole behavioral change—which too often meets resistance—MI is a true instance of give-and-take, in which the interviewer probes for underlying desires and goals, in the hope of pointing out conflicts between continuing current behavioral patterns and the efforts needed to change those patterns. The idea is that the client herself will do a better job of identifying obstacles and ambivalence than will an outside therapist. MI follows steps for working through choices needed to enact change and then *planning* for meaningful change.

In STAND, the clinician uses information gained from MI to help both teens with ADHD and their parents sustain behavior change. Specifically, STAND involves modules related to making plans for conquering homework, providing organization "checks" for the teens with ADHD, emphasizing time-management strategies and study skills, and furthering problem-solving abilities. Hour-long after-school sessions convey the specific skill-building strategies that are used. Again, the format is designed to engage both teens and their parents in mutual problem solving, including the setting up of contracts.

> *By using motivational interviewing, the STAND program acknowledges and capitalizes on teenagers' desire to take control of their own decisions.*

Medications

Because ADHD was not recognized as lasting through adolescence throughout most of the 20th century, there are fewer studies of medications for teens with ADHD than for children with ADHD. But such research is growing, and it shows the same kinds of positive responses to medication for teens as for children. Overall, stimulant medications, and the alternative nonstimulants (see Chapter 6), show benefit for a clear majority of teens who receive them.

In other words, many adolescents who take medication for their ADHD experience increased focus and resistance to distraction, a greater sense of intrinsic motivation, and reductions in impulsive and even dangerous behavioral patterns. Side effects are quite similar to those experienced in childhood as well—with most being manageable and tolerable when the doctor is responsive in terms of needed dosage adjustments.

Why, then, does teens' enthusiasm for continuing to take such medications—even when the pills have helped during childhood—tend to take a real nose-dive during adolescence?

Medication Noncompliance in Teens

Rates of taking ADHD medication fall off dramatically from middle school into high school. This is a particular problem if your daughter is prescribed medication but may now be motivated to give it or sell it to peers. Why, and what can be done about it?

1. Teenagers with ADHD often believe that their having an "illness," which requires them to take pills, is quite off-putting to their peers. All teens tend to be ultraconcerned about what their peers think of them, and there's a stigma attached to being too different from one's peer group. Who are you if you're not a "normal" preteen or teen, like everyone else? If your daughter felt rejected by her peers during childhood, her adolescent years are likely to

magnify her sensitivity to being seen as "different"—especially if she carries with her a form of mental illness.

2. Many teens come to believe that the enhanced focus related to (particularly) taking stimulants may actually be decreasing their spontaneity and creativity. "I feel dull, not myself," many adolescents will say when they take their medication dosage. Or "I feel like I'm in a kind of daze." Perhaps the increased body awareness and general self-awareness that comes with adolescence fuels such self-scrutiny. And what teen doesn't want to feel like her true self (as opposed to being a "zombie" on ADHD meds)—when with her peers or trying to be creative? The same self-awareness may also lead teens to experience common side effects (for example, low appetite, stomachaches, headaches) as more noxious than was the case when they were younger.

Also, when stimulants interfere with sleep, which can happen when doses aren't optimally timed, it can be a real problem for teens. Moreover, adolescents are natural "experimenters," often motivated to see if they still really need the medicine—but often lacking the self-awareness to understand negative consequences if and when they do stop.

3. A number of adolescents may come to rebel against the idea that their parents, and their doctors, know better than they do themselves about their cognition, mood, and behavior. Refusing to take medication may thus be an act of independence, if not defiance—two traits that are the hallmark of the teen years for a great number of adolescents, especially many teens with ADHD.

4. Teens gradually embark on greater responsibilities than previously—and one such responsibility may be to take their medication without their parent handing them the pill or nagging them about it. But ADHD is linked to poor self-monitoring and forgetfulness, even without the defiance of parental control noted just above. Either way, the medication may be left in the pill bottle. Similarly, adolescents with ADHD are typically slower to learn the habit of health routines than their peers are.

> *Be prepared for your daughter to take ADHD medication far less consistently—if at all—than during childhood.*

In sum, for all of the reasons noted above, and probably more, only a small minority of teens with ADHD treated with medication as children continue to take the medications after early to mid-adolescence. And even those who do are often likely to take the medication far less consistently than prescribed. The frequent result is that at the times that your daughter may benefit most from a proper dose of the correct ADHD medication, given the onslaught of challenges related to adolescence, she is increasingly likely to reject taking it (or may take it quite inconsistently).

What to do?

Encouraging Medication Compliance in Your Daughter

As noted in the section on behavioral family therapy with adolescents, an emphasis on collaboration and the family contract could be of real value here. That is, engage your daughter in active conversation about what she perceives as both the potential benefits and the potential liabilities of continuing to take ADHD medication. Even more, as aptly stated by experts on medication for adolescents with ADHD, starting an off-medication trial during middle school or high school can be a real learning experience. (*Note:* Do *not* ask your doctor to engage in one at the beginning of the school year, if the medication was working well the previous school year, and *not* at a time of crisis.) Such a trial can be an excellent means of (1) ascertaining whether medication is actually still needed—or if a dosage adjustment is in order—and (2) engaging your teen actively in the decision-making process. Through parent ratings, teacher ratings, and self-ratings collected both before and during the off-medication period, your daughter and family can be "scientists" engaging in active inquiry about what works best for her. Clearly, it is optimal to engage in such before she begins to question whether medication is worth it.

In addition, the variety of testimonials from celebrities and athletes, the numerous YouTube clips, and other models of adolescents and adults who have done well on medication can be a model and source of inspiration.

Diversion

Finally, I need to bring up the topic of *diversion.* This refers to the use of another person's prescription medication by an individual who does not have a diagnosis or prescription herself. There's been a lot of information about high-school and college students who do not have ADHD but who "borrow" or buy stimulants from someone who does. And, in tandem, those teens and young adults who have been diagnosed with ADHD and have been prescribed medications but who decide to give away or sell the pills instead. In short, the rates are alarmingly high.

Reasons? One is to help enhance late-night study skills or test scores of the individual without ADHD. More nefariously, another reason is to abuse the pills (stimulants can give a "high" and, in the wrong hands, can be quite addictive). Along these lines, among late teens and early adults, one use of stimulants is to be able to keep drinking more alcohol without passing out at parties, because the stimulant will keep the person more alert. Clearly, all this is extremely dangerous territory.

Such diversion is illegal—a felony, actually. Critical research findings show that the supposed benefits of copping someone else's stimulants as "smart pills" or grade-enhancers are highly overrated. In fact, although stimulants can keep people without ADHD up later at night to study, there is no evidence that they actually increase learning (even though the people taking them believe that they are learning more). So, it's an illusion that the medications actually promote better cognitive performance. And, whereas teens and young adults with ADHD are not at all likely to get addicted to their prescribed stimulants, those without ADHD—to whom the pills may get diverted—have a substantial risk of becoming dependent on these medications. The results can be downright dangerous. (*Note:* Nonstimulant ADHD medications are not potent attention boosters and are not potentially addictive, so little or no potential diversion exists for them.)

One of the core reasons for diversion is the large numbers of high-school and college students who continue to get ADHD medications prescribed for themselves but who, for the reasons discussed above, resist them and then stop taking them. The doctors who prescribe such medications need to be extremely careful regarding high-school and college students with ADHD. Clear information on the penalties for selling one's own prescribed ADHD medications to others should be fully available. New research from Brooke Molina of the University of Pittsburgh on means of preventing such diversion reveals that engaging primary-care doctors in the effort to monitor stimulant prescriptions for teens with ADHD can be a starting point.

Heading Off Adult Problems and Negative Outcomes in Adolescence

For girls with ADHD, several key factors and processes can occur during adolescence that predict subsequent impairments and negative outcomes in adulthood. Most of the information below on such factors emanates from my team's BGALS project.

The Development of Other Psychological Problems

Early in this book, I categorized psychological problems that sometimes develop in teens and adults with ADHD as either externalizing issues (such as aggression, delinquency, or substance abuse) or internalizing issues (such as social withdrawal, anxiety, or depression). Both types can present real problems for many domains of life. But it turns out that those two categories are not as separate as might initially be thought. Indeed, it's often individuals who experience both "acting out" behaviors (such as aggression) and "acting in" behaviors (such as anxiety and depression) who have crucial issues with adjusting to adulthood.

In the BGALS, which has spanned childhood through the sample's mid-to-late 20s, we identified two adolescent factors that helped to explain this phenomenon:

- Poor academic achievement in middle school and early high school, which led to school failure and dropout by late adolescence
- Poor self-control and poor ability to delay gratification

Thus, doing whatever you can to keep your daughter engaged in school and in academics—including, as I hammered home earlier in this chapter, identifying key strengths in her to reinforce (even if those may not be in traditional academic subjects)—is crucial. At the same time, engaging her through home contracts that focus on organization and assignment completion (so that small steps lead to success in larger tasks and projects) is also important. So is seeking the kinds of organizational and homework skills programs described above, which may help her to develop greater levels of motivation, along with the ability to reward herself incrementally for a larger payoff later on.

Unplanned Pregnancies and Intimate Partner Violence

You may recall that, in BGALS, nearly 43% of the girls with childhood ADHD had experienced at least one unplanned pregnancy by their mid-20s, contrasted to under 11% of the typically developing comparison sample. Clearly, this is a huge difference. In a systematic examination of adolescent factors that helped to explain such high risk, we examined several potentially important processes, discovering that (1) *academic underachievement* and (2) *engagement in substance use* were crucial in early- to mid-adolescence. Specifically, these were the two factors on the pathway to late-adolescent risky sexual behavior—and subsequently to unplanned pregnancy. In a head-to-head comparison, it was academic underachievement that was the stronger of the two predictors.

The clear message: *Do what you can to keep your daughter academically engaged and supported—and monitor her carefully enough to stop engagement in the abuse of alcohol and illicit substances if at all possible.* Doing so is not easy, given the multiple teachers and subjects in school during those years and given the major temptations of drugs for girls who may not be as socially and academically engaged as others.

Indeed, preventing substance use and abuse is a weighty topic. First, the more academically engaged your daughter is, from elementary school through secondary school, the less likely she is to resort to drugs as a coping mechanism. Second, peer relationships are critical. For girls with ADHD who have been rejected or ignored by many peers, there has been less of a chance to learn and practice important social skills. So, some girls with ADHD may resort to hanging out with girls without strong academic motivation—who may believe that drug use is an excellent coping mechanism.

During adolescence, as in childhood, the presence of one or more friends with strong academic identification and low engagement in substance abuse can be a major protective factor. Encouraging strengths (as emphasized earlier in the chapter) and helping to promote the kinds of activities that engender positive peer support are important.

Girls with ADHD also have a far higher risk for experiencing *intimate partner violence* (verbal or physical attacks by a romantic partner) than do typically developing girls. Again, *low academic performance* in adolescence was the key factor on the pathway to this highly negative outcome. As noted above, keeping your daughter's academic skills and engagement alive—and doing the kind of double duty to keep her secondary school alert to her issues—are of the essence. So is keeping an active dialogue open about her friendships and relationships. Having ADHD does not automatically predict such completely unwelcome and harmful behavior, but there are clear ways to help head it off.

Self-Injury and Suicidal Behavior

In Chapter 8 I pointed out childhood predictors of NSSI and actual suicidal behavior. Additional research has enabled the BGALS team to identify several factors that occur *during adolescence* that may also lead to self-harm by early adulthood:

- *Internalizing problems* (especially depression), which predict suicidal actions, and *externalizing problems* (aggressive behavior), which predict NSSI (like cutting)
- *Peer rejection*, which predicts suicidal behavior, and *peer victimization* (such as being bullied either verbally or physically), which predicts NSSI
- *Physical or sexual abuse* (starting in childhood or adolescence), which predicts suicidal behavior

All of these are potentially important targets for intervention during adolescence. Here are some measures you can take:

- Make sure that the clinician who evaluated your daughter and the professionals who are managing her treatment are well aware of her comorbid conditions and work to treat them.
- Continue to promote your daughter's positive self-image by tapping into her strengths and intrinsic interests and rewarding harder tasks. And even though you can't choose her friends for her, you can make interactions at home as positive as possible and even try to ensure that your daughter has at least one high-quality friend. That friendship can go a long way toward protecting her from being bullied or rejected by other peers. At home, working to keep her engaged in conversation about her choice of friends and partners can go a long way.
- The more you can do to remove your daughter from situations involving any kind of frank abuse, and to get her therapeutic treatment to deal with the after-effects if she has been involved, the better.
- Remember, all of us (including your daughter) can learn from difficult experiences, can learn to prevent getting into similar circumstances, and can come to understand that, with a more optimistic outlook, life can feel far more positive.

Overall, I have presented a lot of information in this chapter. There's no doubt that the preteen and teen years can be challenging, to say the least, particularly when a family has a daughter experiencing ADHD. Indeed, some of the tasks before you are not easy: (1) avoiding the invalidation of your daughter when she's giving you and the family a hard time, (2) coordinating home–school programs across the "wilds" of the multiple teachers of middle school and high school, (3) negotiating contracts when parent and daughter don't always see eye to eye, and (4) promoting clear and positive limits as opposed to coercive interchanges. Still, the overriding message is one of hope and potential change. If you can . . .

- see your daughter for who she is,
- promote strengths as well as focus on areas needing development,
- spend the time and effort to negotiate a viable contract (one that includes meaningful rewards, often based on her interests and strengths),
- get her involved in excellent organizational skills programs, and
- turn your mindset into one of problem solving rather than catastrophizing and self-blaming

. . . then your daughter and the whole family can begin to truly thrive.

TEN

Looking Ahead

I have dedicated this book to helping your daughter thrive, despite ADHD and despite the "triple bind" that continues to negatively influence girls in our society today. If you have applied its information and advice, your daughter may be doing well—or at least better than before you knew how to help her—and your stress levels may have dropped, with family life a bit more tranquil and productive. Maybe your daughter is truly thriving. But what might lie ahead, beyond childhood and adolescence, for your daughter as she enters adulthood?

Throughout this book I've highlighted some of the difficult impairments and life outcomes that many girls with ADHD experience as they mature. The science is progressing enough that researchers and clinicians are getting to a clearer picture in this regard. In particular, some of the most frequent and difficult long-range outcomes are continued academic and organizational problems, including poor time management; high rates of unplanned pregnancy and the experience of intimate partner violence; engagement in self-harm, involving both NSSI and suicidal behavior; and vocational and relationship instability. But my aim here is not just to provide statistics, which speak to group averages. Instead, I want to provide a broad set of perspectives on potential life outcomes for girls with ADHD, emphasizing the following key points for parents and family members:

- Find the right environments and settings in which girls with ADHD may "fit" and thrive as they develop
- Emphasize strengths and find ways of nurturing and supporting such areas of high interest
- Encourage growing independence—but with lifelines and safety nets in place for as long as can be managed
- Forge a realistic yet optimistic mindset about your daughter's future

When you think about overall findings from research, it's essential to remember that each individual is different. This principle clearly applies to girls with ADHD. Any research findings that point to "average" or "expected" outcomes are bound to be misleading for a large number of individuals, especially given the huge variations in genes, early life experiences, parenting and schooling, community resources, and tendencies toward resilience across girls with ADHD as they mature. As we take a look ahead, therefore, your core job will be to balance *realism,* regarding the traits and behavior patterns your daughter brings to the world, with *hope and resolve,* given that there may well be both expected and unexpected ways in which you and your family— and the community supports you gather—can promote her paths to thriving. In many respects, the attitudes and behaviors you bring to the table are all-important.

Does ADHD in Girls Always Persist into Adulthood?

First, let's look at some recent scientific findings, pertinent to both boys and girls with ADHD as they grow up, regarding the likelihood that they will continue to meet diagnostic criteria for this condition into adulthood. All this is a far cry from the accumulated wisdom from a few decades ago, when it was firmly believed that so-called hyperactivity was a male-only condition that rarely, if ever, persisted into adolescence, much less adulthood. Accumulated research (mainly with boys, but now including increasingly larger numbers of girls) tells a far different story.

First, in the most comprehensive examination of whether grade-school children with carefully diagnosed ADHD continue to meet criteria for the disorder during both late adolescence and emerging adulthood, through their mid-to-late 20s, clear findings have emerged. For one thing, although at any given time a now-grown child with ADHD either might just reach the criteria for diagnosis or might fall just short, *a number of key life impairments still tend to remain in place.* For another, across repeated assessments between adolescence and adulthood, the primary pattern appeared to be one of *"waxing and waning."* That, is depending on a number of factors—recent successes or failures; ending up for the time being in a "better-fitting" living situation, job, or relationship; better or worse dealings with family members; and the like—the pattern across time looks more like a gently rolling set of waves than any kind of straight line. In short, symptoms remained higher than those of a matched group of children without ADHD, followed over the same time span. Yet whether members of the ADHD sample actually "have" ADHD at any particular time is typically part of an up-and-down pattern.

The bottom line: Whether a child with ADHD grows up to continue to display ADHD is a fluctuating occurrence. (There's also an open question as to how many symptoms are precisely needed to meet criteria for diagnosis over the years, given that rates of hyperactivity and impulsivity tend to go down with maturity.) Overall, prior skills learned as well as current "fit" with one's life choices and life setting predict whether the diagnosis is still "current" at any given time point. Even more, *nearly 90% of the children with ADHD who are now in adulthood continue to display at least some degree of impairment, ranging from mild to quite severe.*

It is important to know that, for this latter finding, featuring the nearly 600 children with ADHD who participated over 25 years ago in the Multimodal Treatment Study of Children with ADHD (MTA), all participants had been diagnosed with ADHD–Combined when they entered the study at ages 7 to 9 years. It is still uncertain, therefore, whether the same would be true for those with ADHD–Inattentive (but remember that inattentive symptoms are more likely to persist into adulthood than are hyperactive symptoms). And the MTA sample was composed of 80% boys. Still, the findings above apply to the 116 girls with ADHD who enrolled in this landmark study.

Second, in my team's BGALS investigation—composed of 140 girls with ADHD as they entered the study, when they were 6–12 years of age— we found parallel trends. This sample included, during childhood, girls with both ADHD–Combined and ADHD–Inattentive. Overall, taking into account the varying cutoff points used to define ADHD in adulthood, a clear majority continued to meet diagnostic criteria. Importantly, even those who no longer consistently met criteria for ADHD by late adolescence and early adulthood still had high rates of unplanned pregnancies, low school achievement, weight gain over time, and objectively rated life problems. (It's also important to note, however, that those girls and young women with the strongest risk for engaging in self-harm and employment problems, overall, were those whose ADHD symptoms persisted over time.) The long and short of it is that, in girls as well as boys, *a number of problematic life outcomes are likely to occur into the period of adulthood, even if particular symptoms are no longer rated by the woman in question, or adults who know her well, as falling in the diagnostic range.*

A couple of important, clear implications of the research evidence are as follows:

- Helping to promote strengths—and to focus on academic, organizational, and time-management skills, along with treatment for comorbid conditions—is a better long-term bet than simply reducing ADHD symptoms.

- Finding the best environments (such as postsecondary schooling, optimal jobs, and positive living situations) that can provide optimal "fit" for your growing daughter with ADHD is crucial.

Keep in mind that ADHD in girls comes with slow maturation, poor self-regulation, and low intrinsic motivation. These problems can make skill building difficult for your daughter, taking a toll on her potential for independence and thriving. On the other hand, most of the studies to date that have followed kids with ADHD into adulthood rely on measures of problems and impairments. As a result, the entire field may be missing out on those girls who do thrive and the kinds of settings and encouragements that can help to promote adaptive functioning.

Promoting Strengths and Compensating for Weaknesses

My own research team has made attempts to identify the protective factors that might be best suited to promote thriving in girls with ADHD as they grow out of childhood and adolescence. Unfortunately, we have not had great success in doing so at any kind of overall level, but our latest round of follow-up into the age range of their 30s may prove quite helpful in this regard. Some of the usual suspects—for example, high intelligence—just don't pan out as protective factors, and a trait such as IQ isn't terribly easy to modify in any event. We did find that friendships in childhood appear to be protective against being victimized by peers. In fact, this protective factor applied to both girls with ADHD and their typically developing agemates.

Also, when parents make shifts in their parenting toward a truly authoritative style—blending warmth and responsiveness with appropriate controls and limit setting—their offspring with ADHD show large gains toward normalization of their symptoms and impairments, particularly when optimal medications are in the picture as well.

Overall, a review of protective factors for youth with ADHD, as they head into the adult years, lands on two core processes:

- Positive parenting
- Social/peer acceptance (meaning that the girl receives at least a modicum of social support, including friendships)

Indeed, a large European study of boys and girls with ADHD during adolescence found that (1) *improvements in family climate* and (2) *social supports* were the core protective factors against the intensification of ADHD symptoms over time.

So, the material from Chapter 5 on parenting, and many of the points in the second half of this book—on behavioral family therapy, contracting, organizational skills, and helping to promote social engagement—are what I'd recommend for you to review. And your real task is to put into practice the hard work involved in making changes in your own attitudes and parenting styles—and engaging schools and treatment providers—that can make a difference.

Yet there is no magic formula, across all girls with ADHD, regarding protection. In fact, what might be a protective factor for one girl with ADHD may well differ from the protective influences for another such girl. In other words, as I highlighted in Chapter 9, *find strengths and positive influences for your own daughter—and nurture them as best you can.* Sometimes, as a parent, you may need to toughen up and hold the line with limits (this is more likely to be the case for a girl with ADHD–Combined, with oppositional tendencies). At other times, however, you may need to back off a bit and see what your daughter is telling you through her behavior: Namely, that she might not fit a "straight and narrow" mold of academic performance and behavioral conformity. Instead, she may thrive in ways that you might never have predicted or expected when she was young.

Approaching this issue from a somewhat different angle, are there career paths that seem to work best for kids with ADHD, particularly girls, as they attain adulthood? Again, there is certainly no single, one-size-fits-all answer. In one important study, interviewers asked probing questions of young adults with ADHD of both sexes. Questions dealt with their own views of what ADHD is, how they experienced the symptoms over time, and what may have been protective influences in their lives. Not surprisingly, participants viewed their symptoms as dependent on the context. That is, in some settings they were better able to focus—but in rote, routine work, they were far less able to focus or self-regulate. Many participants stated that their own characteristic symptoms, including high energy levels, can become strengths versus liabilities. For a number of the participants, tasks and jobs that were somewhat stressful, moderately challenging, novel, hands-on or physically demanding, fast-paced, and intrinsically interesting had led to initial careers of thriving.

Many of these depictions could characterize individuals with the combined form of ADHD, with its often fast-paced style and intense need for activity. For those with the inattentive form, a more reflective, individually paced set of job skills and requirements could be optimal (for example, Kay in Chapter 9, who found solace and commitment in working with animals). The overriding point is that, looking ahead, you should be prepared for some less-than-traditional expectations and roles for your daughter with ADHD as she moves forward on her journey. Alternatively, if she has a hankering for more traditional jobs, she may well need continued supports (such as medication, or the kind of assistance that others typically do) to thrive. It's all part of the evolving set of expectations that you work through, sensitively and carefully, with your daughter. It's never too late to find new options for thriving, as you and she continue to probe the best avenues for success.

What's the Right Outlook? What Can You Do?

Back in Chapter 1, and at several points later in the book, I raised the concepts of *radical acceptance* of and *radical commitment* toward your daughter with ADHD. Both ideas remain important as your daughter matures.

When you learned (or may soon be learning) that your daughter has ADHD, it probably was (or will probably be) a real wallop. *You mean, she has a disability? She'll never be . . . well . . . normal? How have I, or we, failed her? What should our family expect? I'm not sure I'm up to this challenge—look how stressful our lives are at this point.*

As I have highlighted and urged in the previous chapters, it's important to understand that your daughter is likely to be behind other girls in brain maturation, behaving like a girl several years younger than her peers. Some of the problems that come with that lag in development will follow your daughter through adolescence:

- She may not be as well regulated as other girls.
- She may still need external rewards and support beyond what you probably expected when she was born.
- If your daughter continues her education past high school, you may still need to encourage her to obtain college accommodations—and see that she does work to enlist teachers and professors in her staying organized through the difficult material she is encountering.
- You (and she) may need to keep finding experienced professionals in your community to help with her self-regulation and skill attainment.

Crucially, you'll also need to realize that you have never been to blame for all this—ADHD is predominantly a biologically based condition—but that you have plenty of extra responsibility for helping to guide your daughter along paths toward thriving. Furthermore, a lot of that responsibility relates to reconfiguring your parenting style toward a decided blend of high warmth/support and high clarity about limits and controls, as I hope you have been doing through your daughter's childhood and adolescence. You have probably also needed to confront the often-weighty issue of whether she will do best on medications for her condition, on top of behavioral family therapy, CBT, school supports and accommodations, and other treatments for comorbid conditions she may have—needs that may well continue as she matures.

As your daughter has moved from childhood to adolescence, she has needed, more and more, to start carrying the ball. At the same time, you have had to be there for her in new and different ways to scaffold and support her growing attempts at self-regulation. As she nears the age when most individuals are on their own, it's essential to continue following these principles:

- Radically accept your daughter's differences. Some of these differences may have been counter to your initial expectations, hopes, and desires. But especially if she's your biological daughter, you may also have seen some real similarities to your own attentional, self-regulatory, and behavioral tendencies.
- Radically realize that she will need a level of structure and support that many other girls and young women may not. As long as you continue to accept her and relish her differences, your help in structuring her environment can truly help her to thrive, even as an adult.

So, what are the crucial action steps involved? I've covered them in the prior chapters of this book. As a brief, headline-style review, here are the critical points that I emphasize strongly:

1. *Find ways to love and support your daughter, no matter what.* Yes, she may not be precisely whom you expected. Yes, she presents more challenges than the typical child or teen. Yes, you may have crossed over into major parental and family stress many times during her development. But seeing her clearly, cherishing her, relishing her strengths and positive qualities, and finding ways of letting her know how much you care for and support her are at the top of the list. This is your crucial challenge as a parent of a daughter with ADHD.

Continue to look for emerging interests as she becomes a teen and post-teen. Maybe a particular high-school class got her excited; perhaps she has picked up a new hobby or seen, from a peer, a talent she'd like to develop. There are lots of potential options out there, but you and she need to continue to seek them out.

2. *Find ways to engage in appropriate controls and limits as well.* As I've emphasized repeatedly, *the essence of authoritative parenting is the blend of warmth and love with limit setting and supportive control.* Your daughter has undoubtedly tried your patience (perhaps through her inattention and poor self-regulation), and it may sometimes seem that raising her has been a battle of wills (perhaps through her poor impulse control and oppositional nature). You can't cave in, but there's a major cost of being perennially engaged in arguments and screaming bouts. They self-perpetuate, and everyone loses in the end. Reward charts (for younger girls), contracts (for teens), careful monitoring of the safety of the home and of her whereabouts—and the enforcing of clear behavioral limits—are all the name of the game.

The ways you express warmth will, of course, change as she gets older—but there's nothing like heartfelt praise and respect from you at any age. Keep your antennae lifted and look for successes, even mini-successes. And limits will evolve, as well. It may be that, in her moves toward independence, you will need to limit financial support so that she does not remain dependent on you. Or discussions (which too often turn into arguments) about roommates or romantic partners may need to be monitored with a timer. In this age of lowered expectations that our offspring's' incomes may ever match our own, along with the incredibly stressful circumstances that most of us find ourselves in these days, it's difficult to support any young adult's moves toward independence, but particularly so when she's had years of living with ADHD.

3. *Engage her teachers and school.* Chapter 7 featured a number of different strategies regarding both school accommodations and coordination of home and school behavioral programs. As you may have discovered, it takes real work on your part to ensure such coordination, but the end results are clearly worth it. You can continue these kinds of efforts even after high school.

Just in the way that there's no inherently "best" educational option for girls with ADHD in primary or secondary school, as discussed at length in Chapter 7, there's no absolute "must" in terms of college options for young women with ADHD, given the huge differences in personality, style, preference, and aptitude among those who receive the diagnosis. However, it's a good idea to look for colleges with reputations for good services for individuals with learning differences (and all kinds of disabilities, for that matter). See the Resources at the end of this book for suggestions along these lines.

4. *Get high-quality professional help.* From the assessment and diagnostic process all the way through engagement in behavioral family therapy and medication management, it pays to ask around, thoroughly and carefully, to assure that you work with assessors and clinicians with sound knowledge of ADHD in girls. Adult women with ADHD will clearly benefit from the same care.

5. *Engage with other parents and supports.* Seek, in your community, support groups and advocacy groups or other means of engaging with families also experiencing the challenges of raising a daughter with ADHD. It's a hard road to travel alone. Support and encouragement can both keep you engaged and help you navigate routes to community-level programs and supports. You may find yourself benefiting from these resources even into your daughter's adulthood.

6. *Remember that ADHD may not be the only issue your daughter is experiencing.* Getting professional help for her anxiety/depression, learning problems, trauma-related issues, or additional medical and psychological issues is essential. Vigilance here can be particularly helpful as a girl with ADHD becomes a woman with ADHD, with its inevitable greater demands.

It doesn't get any easier, as your daughter matures, to separate out "what's ADHD" from "what's depression . . . or anxiety . . . or PTSD . . . or a continuing learning disorder." So, related to points 4 and 5 above, finding professionals with expertise in adults—particularly women—with ADHD and comorbid disorders is a crucial endeavor. You probably won't find optimal clinicians unless you actively seek them.

7. *Get help for your own levels of stress . . . and potentially, ADHD and depression.* I've emphasized repeatedly that parenting stress and family stress—and even depression—are frequent accompaniments of raising off-spring with ADHD. Moreover, the genetics underlying ADHD are such that a large number of biological parents of youth with this condition will be experiencing parallel issues in organization, time management, and self-regulation. There's no shame in seeking help for yourself along these lines, over and above the behavioral family therapy and other child-focused interventions in which you engage. In fact, it's a sign of strength to seek help for yourself. Everyone can benefit, especially when you've been in this over the long haul.

Too many parents of girls with ADHD expend so much time, effort, and worry about their daughter that they tend to neglect their own stress levels and/or mental health issues. Support groups and advocacy meetings can therefore be helpful not only for locating resources for your daughter but also for yourself. If you're not functioning optimally, no one is going to win.

8. *Reward yourself.* Parenting a girl with ADHD is no easy path. Make sure that you, and those around you, recognize and reward your efforts. Progress may be slow at the beginning, as new habits and parenting practices take time to develop. Plan small (and even larger) rewards for yourself, for both effort and the successes you experience with your daughter, today and in the future.

Friends and relatives can help here, with suggestions of outings, or prebought gifts that get "released" to you, when you've stuck with it for a certain time period or when certain milestones on your daughter's journey are reached. Neglecting yourself can be a ticket for going down with the ship. You deserve recognition, respite, and reward for your efforts.

9. *Realize that our society's straight-and-narrow paths toward "success" can be a killer.* Not everyone has the same behavioral, attention-related, and emotional style! The traits underlying ADHD can be a real liability in traditional classrooms, and disorganization and lack of self-control can make work performance and relationship satisfaction a real challenge in many instances. Yet in the right contexts, and with the right supports, they can also propel out-of-the-box thinking and creative problem solving—and a unique energy. Again,

try to search for and support strengths and provide unique opportunities for your daughter, as you "read" her interests and motivations. We all continue to develop beyond adolescence, and your daughter with ADHD will, too.

The triple bind, from earlier chapters, is real—not only for preteen and teenage girls but also for their family members. It's super-important to examine your values, for yourself and your daughter, and try not to get caught up in unrealistic expectations that end up breeding misery and a sense of helplessness. Your overarching goal is to help her find her *way.*

10. *Keep at it!* Parenting a daughter with ADHD is a marathon, not a sprint. Don't expect major changes overnight. Pace yourself. Realize that with adolescence, both new challenges and new strengths will emerge. You're her parent for the rest of her life, and experiencing the changes in her and in yourself can be a thing of wonder, not just despair.

Overall, with all of this book's material in mind, please embark and continue on the journey with the realization that you're not alone, that there are multiple paths to "success," that the whole family needs to adapt, and that there are a lot of different ways of coping and succeeding in our modern world. Your daughter can thrive with your ongoing help and guidance.

Resources

The following are websites and other resources for families of girls with ADHD. I begin with national-level information sources before highlighting a few of the literally hundreds of books on ADHD, with a focus on those that may be of real use for parents. I conclude with resources found under alphabetically listed topic headings.

Advocacy and Information-Dissemination Organizations (National and International)

Attention Deficit Disorder Association (ADDA) is an international nonprofit organization. focused chiefly on adults with ADHD, designed to support innovation and best practices:
https://add.org

Children and Adults with Attention-Deficit Hyperactivity Disorder (CHADD) is a U.S.-based nonprofit organization dedicated to providing information, support, and advocacy for individuals with ADHD:
https://chadd.org/about

ADHD Australia is a nonprofit organization, in Australia, which aims to promote dissemination of evidence-based practices and reduce ADHD-related stigma:
www.adhdaustralia.org.au/about-us-info

ADHD Ireland is a nonprofit organization based in Ireland, designed to promote resources, information, and networking related to ADHD:
https://adhdireland.ie

ADHD New Zealand is a nonprofit organization based in New Zealand, designed to support and connect individuals and families living with ADHD to relevant resources:
www.adhd.org.nz/about-us.html

ADHD UK is a charity designed by people with ADHD to support others with ADHD:
https://adhduk.co.uk/support

CADDRA is a nonprofit research organization in Canada that promotes evidence-based assessment and treatment guidelines for ADHD, sponsors conferences, and promotes cross-province collaborations. It is comprehensive and state-of-the-art:
www.caddra.ca

Health Navigator New Zealand presents clear facts about ADHD:
www.healthnavigator.org.nz/health-a-z/a/adhd-children

Open Forest is a mental health and coaching organization, with articles on a range of mental-health topics, including ADHD:
https://openforest.net

Key Books

Seemingly countless books on ADHD are available, ranging from dense academic treatises to easy-to-read self-help books. The following 10 were published in recent years and rely on strong scientific backing—yet are general enough and sufficiently readable to be of use to readers of this book, also including clinicians.

Barkley, R. A. (2020). *Taking charge of ADHD: The complete, authoritative guide for parents* (4th ed.). New York: Guilford Press. [Fourth edition of immensely popular guide for parents of girls and boys with ADHD.]

Barkley, R. A. (2022). *Treating ADHD in children and adolescents: What every clinician needs to know.* New York: Guilford Press. [Handbook for pediatricians, child and adolescent psychologists, clinical psychologists, school psychologists, social workers, and more, with up-to-date information on evaluation and treatment procedures. More advanced and clinically focused than *Taking Charge of ADHD* but still quite readable.]

Chronis-Tuscano, A., O'Brien, K., & Danko, C. (2021). *Supporting caregivers of children with ADHD.* New York: Oxford University Press. [Handbook mainly for clinicians on how to assess and treat parents and other caregivers of youth with ADHD, particularly if they have mental-health conditions themselves. Although the text is somewhat technical, parents can benefit from this information.]

DuPaul, G. J., & Stoner, G. (2014). *ADHD in the schools: Assessment and intervention strategies* (3rd ed.). New York: Guilford Press. [Third edition of a book designed mainly for school teachers and professionals, on educational evaluation and intervention for youth with ADHD. Good information for parents as well.]

Hinshaw, S. P., & Ellison, K. (2015). *ADHD: What everyone needs to know.* New York: Oxford University Press. [An easy-to-read book in "Question and Answer" format on multiple aspects of ADHD, written for families and the lay public.]

Hinshaw, S. P., & Scheffler, R. M. (2014). *The ADHD explosion: Myths, medication, money, and today's push for performance.* New York: Oxford University Press. [Trade book, written for both the lay public and professionals/policy makers, on the realities of ADHD in the 21st century.]

Miller, K. (2018). *Thriving with ADHD workbook for kids.* Emeryville, CA: Althea Press. [A cleverly designed and written, information-filled but basic workbook for youth with ADHD as well as their families.]

Nadeau, K. G., Littman, E. B., & Quinn, P. O. (2015). *Understanding girls with ADHD: How they feel and why they do what they do* (2nd ed.). Washington, DC: Advantage Books. [Second edition of information-laden book on girls with ADHD, focusing on differences from boys.]

Saline, S. (2018). *What your ADHD child wishes you knew: Working together to empower kids for success in school and life.* New York: Tarcherperigee. [Book for parents, written at a basic yet compelling level, on the experience of ADHD from an offspring's perspective.]

Tyler, A. K. (2021). *Raising a girl with ADHD: A practical guide to help girls harness their unique strengths and abilities.* Emeryville: Rockridge Press. [Another parent-friendly book focusing on practical strategies to empower girls with ADHD.]

For an alternate listing, see *ADDitude Magazine*'s "10 Books that Every Parent Should Read" (although the listing includes 11!). Only two of these 11 overlap with the 10 references above:
https://additudemag.com/slideshows/parenting-books-about-adhd-and-ld

Specific Websites and Resources by Topic

Accommodations

Excellent source on basic classroom practices and accommodations, from the U.S. Centers for Disease Control and Prevention:
https://cdc.gov/ncbddd/adhd/school-success.html

Another clear and readable source on basic classroom adjustments and accommodations, from the advocacy group Children and Adults with ADHD (CHADD):
https://chadd.org/for-educators/classroom-accommodations

A clear set of 20 basic accommodations for ADHD, from *ADDitude Magazine:*
https://additudemag.com/20-adhd-accommodations-that-work

Assessment and Diagnosis

A helpful WebMD website posting on ratings scales for helping to diagnose ADHD in children:
https://webmd.com/add-adhd/childhood-adhd/adhd-rating-scales

A list of tests and assessments for diagnosing ADHD, also from WebMD:
https://webmd.com/add-adhd/childhood-adhd/adhd-tests-making-assessment

From *ADDitude Magazine,* a thorough article on dos and don'ts for an ADHD diagnostic assessment: "Your Complete ADHD Diagnosis and Testing Guide":
https://additudemag.com/adhd-testing-diagnosis-guide

Behavioral Family Therapy (and Beyond)

Parent–Child Interaction Therapy (PCIT): See the website for the organization PCIT International:
www.pcit.org

An excellent, parent-focused book for children with disruptive problems is the following: Barkley, R. A., & Benton, C. M. (2013). *Your defiant child: Eight steps to better behavior* (2nd ed.). New York: Guilford Press.

From the University of Maryland, the Stroud Foundation, and CHADD, a series of videos on the teaching of evidence-based practices for youth with ADHD:
https://chadd.org/stroud-umdadhdtools

Colleges with Resources for Students with ADHD

From the Child Mind Institute, an article on colleges and tips for students with ADHD:
https://childmind.org/article/10-tips-going-college-ADHD

From Verywellmind, "Choosing a College When You Have ADHD":
https://verywellmind.com/choosing-a-college-when-you-have-adhd-20565

From CHADD, "Selecting and Applying to Colleges for Students with ADHD":
https://chadd.org/wp-content/uploads/2018/05/CollegeandADHD_ApplyingtoCollege.pdf

Daily Report Cards

Clear report from *ADDitude Magazine,* which includes a free download of a template for a DRC home–school system:
https://additudemag.com/daily-report-card-to-improve-adhd-classroom-behavior

From Verywellmind, "Daily Report Cards to Improve a Child's ADHD Behavior":
https://verywellmind.com/how-to-use-a-daily-report-card-20840

Girls and Women with ADHD

From *ADDitude Magazine,* an article titled "The Best Web Resources for Women with ADHD," with links to 10 different websites:
https://additudemag.com/best-web-resources-for-adhd-women

From WebMD, "ADHD in Women and Girls":
https://webmd.com/add-adhd/ss/slideshow-adhd-women-girls

From Verywellmind, "20 Signs and Symptoms of ADHD in Girls":
https://verywellmind.com/adhd-in-girls-symptoms-of-adhd-in-girls-20547

From ADHD expert Ellen Littman, "Girls with ADHD Face Unique Challenges":
www.smartkidswithld.org/getting-help/adhd/girls-with-adhd-face-unique-challenges

Low-Income Families/Children of Color

A wonderful article and video, based on research from Boston Medical Center, describing different stages of engagement in the ADHD evaluation and treatment process for families with limited resources:
https://healthcity.bmc.org/population-health/6-stages-engagement-framework-may-help-better-treat-children-adhd

Medications

An extremely clear and thorough chart of medications in common use for the treatment of ADHD, from Northwell Health. *Note:* When you open the link, click on the blue oval just over halfway down the page ("I Have Read the End User Agreement and Agree")—and the two-page chart will open.
www.ADHDMedicationGuide.com

Also listed in Further Reading for Chapter 8, the following book is extremely helpful:

Wilens, T. E., & Hammerness, P. G. (2016). *Straight talk about psychiatric medications for kids* (4th ed.). New York: Guilford Press.

Organizations Dealing with Comorbid Conditions

From Mentalhealth.gov, a listing of organizations dealing with many different kinds of child and adolescent mental health conditions:
https://mentalhealth.gov/talk/community-conversation

From Child Mind Institute, an informative set of informational guidelines and treatment resources for a wide range of child and adolescent mental health conditions:
https://childmind.org/care

Depression/Anxiety

See the website of the Centers for Disease Control and Prevention, under child mental health:
https://cdc.gov/childrensmentalhealth/depression.html

See also the website of the Anxiety and Depression Association of America (ADAA):
https://adaa.org

And see the website of the HEARD Alliance:
www.heardalliance.org (see especially the tab for "Resources")

Posttraumatic Stress Disorder and Trauma in General

See the website of the National Child Traumatic Stress Network:
https://nctsn.org/what-is-child-trauma

Bipolar Disorder

See the information-laden website from Boston Children's Hospital:
https://childrenshospital.org/conditions/bipolar-disorder

Also, see the website tab from Mental Health America:
https://mhanational.org/bipolar-disorder-children

Learning Disorders

See the comprehensive website of the Learning Disabilities Association of America:
https://ldaamerica.org

And the site for the National Center for Learning Disabilities:
https://ncld.org

Youth Suicide and Self-Harm

See the website, with a key list of resources (plus a toolkit) from Zero Suicide:
https://zerosuicide.edc.org/resources/populations/children-and-youth

See also the comprehensive website of the JED Foundation:
https://jedfoundation.org

Parenting Styles and Practices

A good summary of authoritative parenting, as applied to ADHD, from *ADDitude Magazine:*
https://additudemag.com/authoritative-parenting-discipline-adhd-kids

An interview with ADHD expert Kathleen Nadeau, "Raising Girls with ADHD":
https://chadd.org/attention-article/raising-girls-with-adhd

From Australia, two websites, one on raising grade-school-aged children with ADHD and the other on raising adolescents with ADHD:
https://raisingchildren.net.au/school-age/development/adhd/managing-adhd-5-11-years
https://raisingchildren.net.au/teens/development/adhd/managing-adhd-12-18-years

Also from Australia, from the Royal Children's Hospital of Melbourne:
www.rch.org.au/kidsinfo/fact_sheets/ADHD_ways_to_help_children_with_ADHD

Role Models of Individuals with ADHD

From YouTube, a video of 10 inspirational "role models" of individuals with histories of ADHD, including Adam Levine, Channing Tatum, Justin Timberlake, and Michael Phelps:
www.youtube.com/watch?v=E6LxfDFSZ0s

From Edge Foundation, "Simone Biles—The Heart and Soul of a Champion":
https://edgefoundation.org/simone-biles-the-heart-and-soul-of-a-champion

From YouTube, "Women and Girls with ADHD":
www.youtube.com/watch?v=aRngPNeLxEM

From *ADDitude Magazine*, "5 Women with ADHD Who Are Changing the Conversation":
https://additudemag.com/adhd-success-stories-women-with-add

Schools and School-Based Interventions

Article from *ADDitude Magazine*, "10 Ways We Would Fix the U.S. School System":
https://additudemag.com/slideshows/how-can-we-improve-education-for-students-with-adhd

Workbook from ADHD expert Russell Barkley:
Managing ADHD in School: The Best Evidence-Based Methods for Teachers, published in
    2016 by PESI, Inc. (see also Further Reading for Chapter 7)

Social Skills

Fact-filled guide on enhancing social skills for children with ADHD, from Verywellmind:
https://verywellmind.com/how-to-improve-social-skills-in-children-with-adhd-20727

Treatments Beyond Core Evidence-Based Treatments

By "beyond" I mean treatments other than behavioral family therapy, CBT, social skills interventions, and medications.

See Appendix D of Barkley, R. A. (2022). *Treating ADHD in children and adolescents: What every clinician needs to know.* New York: Guilford Press. Appendix D is titled "Unproven and Disproven Treatments for ADHD."

Aerobic Exercise: From *ADDitude Magazine,* see "The ADHD Exercise Solution," which reveals evidence that exercise can in fact supplement the core evidence-based treatments:
https://additudemag.com/the-adhd-exercise-solution

Organizational Skills: See the book-length accounts in Gallagher, R., Abikoff, H. B., & Spira, E. G. (2014). *Organizational skills training for children with ADHD: An empirically supported treatment.* New York: Guilford Press.

Neurofeedback: The most recent, highly controlled research shows that neurofeedback does not produce greater benefits for ADHD symptoms than "false" neurofeedback, for which the feedback to the youth with ADHD is not actually attuned to her or his brainwave patterns:
www.elsevier.com/about/press-releases/research-and-journals/benefits-of-neurofeedback-for-those-with-adhd-mainly-due-to-factors-other-than-brainwave-training

Specific Cognitive Training: See, from *ADDitude Magazine,* "Brain Training for ADHD: What Is It? Does It Work?"—the article reveals that effects are far from clear or strong:
https://additudemag.com/adhd-brain-training-neurofeedback-memory

Video Games and Apps: See, from *ADDitude Magazine,* "Like a Personal Trainer for Your Brain," which reveals the promise—and the lack of applicability to real-world outcomes—of tech-based solutions related to ADHD:
https://additudemag.com/slideshows/brain-training-apps-like-lumosity

Trauma-Informed Care

Learning about trauma-informed care may be particularly important if your daughter was adopted or in foster care or otherwise has an abuse history.

Thorough website from the Trauma-Informed Care Resource Implementation Center:
https://traumainformedcare.chcs.org

Another excellent website from the U.S. Substance Abuse and Mental Health Services Administration (SAMHSA):
https://samhsa.gov/childrens-awareness-day/past-events/2018/child-traumatic-stress-resources

And another, from the National Child Traumatic Stress Network:
https://nctsn.org/trauma-informed-care

The National Child Traumatic Stress Network (NCTSN) lists Parent–Child Interaction Therapy specifically under one of its tabs:
https://nctsn.org/interventions/parent-child-interaction-therapy

Treatment Modalities for Comorbid Conditions

From Verywellmind, see:
https://verywellmind.com/what-is-cognitive-behavior-therapy-2795747

Dialectical Behavior Therapy

From WebMD, see:
https://webmd.com/mental-health/dialectical-behavioral-therapy

From Verywellmind, see:
https://verywellmind.com/dialectical-behavior-therapy-1067402

Oppositional Defiant Disorder

See this excellent article from *ADDitude Magazine:* "Why Is My Child So Angry?":
https://addmdmag.com/adhd-odd-why-is-my-child-angry

Autism Spectrum Disorder

See, from the Centers for Disease Control and Prevention:
https://cdc.gov/ncbddd/autism/treatment.html

Substance Use Disorders

See the thorough overview from the Agency for Healthcare Research and Quality:
https://effectivehealthcare.ahrq.gov/products/substance-use-disorders-adolescents/protocol

Further Reading

For each chapter, I provide 10–14 key sources, including books, book chapters, and research articles, as background material for the text. Some of the most general of these references appear for multiple chapters. If this were an academically oriented book, there would over 50 references for each chapter! Indeed, the scientific literature on ADHD is growing at ever-faster rates. Still, readers interested in deeper reading can certainly check out the reference section in each of the entries below, to gain a wider network of sources.

Chapter 1: What Does ADHD Look Like in Girls?

American Psychiatric Association. (2013). *Diagnostic and statistical manual of mental disorders* (5th ed.). Arlington, VA: American Psychiatric Press. [Includes the official U.S. diagnostic criteria for ADHD.]

Angold, A., Costello, E. J., & Erkanli, A. (1999). Comorbidity. *Journal of Child Psychology and Psychiatry, 40,* 57–87. [Classic article on comorbidity in child and adolescent psychiatry.]

Barkley, R. A. (Ed.). (2015). *Attention deficit hyperactivity disorder: A handbook for diagnosis and treatment* (4th ed.). New York: Guilford Press. [Major handbook comprising multiple chapters, each by experts in the field, on crucial aspects of ADHD.]

Barkley, R. A. (2022). *Treating ADHD in children and adolescents: What every clinician needs to know.* New York: Guilford Press. [Authoritative guide on assessment and treatment of ADHD, written for clinicians but with valuable information for parents.]

Beery, A. K., & Zucker, I. (2011). Sex bias in neuroscience and biomedical research. *Neuroscience & Biobehavioral Reviews, 35,* 565–572. [Classic article on male predominance in not only human research but also animal research.]

Cenat, J. M., Blais-Rochette, C., Morse, C., Vandette, M. P., Noorishad, P. G., Kogan, C., . . . Labelle, P. R. (2021). Prevalence and risk factors associated with attention-deficit/hyperactivity disorder among US Black individuals: A systematic review and meta-analysis. *JAMA Psychiatry, 78,* 21–28. [Important review article revealing rise in diagnosis of ADHD in Black individuals in recent years.]

Danielson, M. L., Bitsko, R. H., Ghandour, R. M., Holbrook, J. R., Kogan, M. D., & Blumberg, S. J. (2018). Prevalence of parent reported ADHD diagnosis and associated treatment among U.S. children and adolescents, 2016. *Journal of Clinical Child and Adolescent Psychology, 47,* 199–212. [National data from large parent survey in U.S. on diagnosed prevalence of ADHD in boys and girls.]

Goodman, S. H., Lahey, B. B., Fielding, B., Dulcan, M., Narrow, W., & Regier, D. (1997). Representativeness of clinical samples of youths with mental disorders: A preliminary population-based study. *Journal of Abnormal Psychology, 106,* 3–14. [Scientific article on the topic of how samples of clinically referred children differ substantially from representative samples of children.]

Hinshaw, S. P., Nguyen, N. T., O'Grady, S. M., & Rosenthal, E. A. (2022). ADHD in girls and women: Underrepresentation, longitudinal processes, and key directions. *Journal of Child Psychology and Psychiatry, Annual Research Review, 63,* 484–496. [Review of historical trends related to the underrecognition of ADHD in girls and women, as well as accumulated research on girls and women with ADHD.]

Hinshaw, S. P., & Scheffler, R. M. (2014). *The ADHD explosion: Myths, medication, money, and today's push for performance.* New York: Oxford University Press. [Comprehensive book on controversies related to ADHD, myths and realities of ADHD, and influence of state-by-state testing policies on greatly differing rates of ADHD diagnoses within the United States.]

Quinn, P. O., & Madhoo, M. (2014). A review of attention deficit/hyperactivity disorder in women and girls: Uncovering this hidden diagnosis. *The Primary Care Companion for CNS Disorders, 16,* PCC.13r01596. [Article on differences between male versus female form of ADHD and how to detect ADHD optimally in females.]

Wolraich, M. L., Hagan, J. F., Allan, C., Chan, E., Davison, D., Earls, M., . . . Zurhellen, W. (2019). Clinical practice guideline for the diagnosis, evaluation, and treatment of attention-deficit/hyperactivity disorder in children and adolescents. *Pediatrics, 144,* e20192528. [The official practice guidelines for ADHD's diagnosis and treatment, from the American Academy of Pediatrics.]

Young, S., Adamo, N., Asgeirsdottir, B. B., Branney, P., Beckett, M., Colley, W., . . . Woodhouse, E. (2020). Females with ADHD: An expert consensus statement taking a lifespan approach providing guidance for the identification and treatment of attention-deficit/hyperactivity disorder in girls and women. *BMC Psychiatry, 20,* 404. [Authoritative British review article on manifestations of ADHD in girls and women.]

Chapter 2: Does Your Daughter Have ADHD?

American Psychiatric Association. (2013). *Diagnostic and statistical manual of mental disorders* (5th ed.). Arlington, VA: Author. [Includes the official U.S. diagnostic criteria for ADHD.]

Banachewski, T., Coghill, D., & Zuddas, A. (Eds.). (2018). *Oxford textbook of attention deficit hyperactivity disorder.* London: Oxford University Press. [Excellent compendium, from a largely non-U.S. perspective, including chapters on assessment and diagnosis.]

Barkley, R. A. (2022). *Treating ADHD in children and adolescents: What every clinician needs to know.* New York: Guilford Press. [Authoritative guide on multiple aspects of ADHD, written for clinicians but with valuable information for parents. For information on comorbid conditions, see especially Chapter 4. For information on parental reactions to their offspring's diagnosis with ADHD, see Chapter 5.]

Becker, S. P. (Ed.). (2020). *ADHD in adolescents: Development, assessment, and treatment.* New York: Guilford Press. [Edited book with excellent range of chapters on ADHD during the teen years. For assessment of teens, see Chapter 13, by DuPaul et al.; see also Chapter 9, by Becker and Fogleman.]

Brown, T. E. (Ed.). (2009). *ADHD comorbidities: Handbook for ADHD complications in children and adults.* Washington, DC: American Psychiatric Press. [Important compilation of chapters on comorbid conditions that exist alongside ADHD.]

DuPaul, G. J., & Stoner, G. (2014). *ADHD in the schools: Assessment and intervention strategies* (3rd ed.). New York: Guilford Press. [Excellent book, with chapters focused on assessment, treatment planning, collaboration with professionals, and the like.]

Meyer, B. J., Stevenson, J., & Sonuga-Barke, E. (2020). Sex differences in the meaning of parent and teacher ratings of ADHD behaviors: An observational study. *Journal of Attention Disorders, 24,* 1847–1856. [Research article revealing that adult ratings of ADHD symptoms in children appear to be biased in terms of underrepresenting girls.]

Norvilitis, J. M. (Ed.). (2015). *ADHD: New directions in diagnosis and treatment.* Rijeka, Croatia: InTech Open. [Comprehensive edited textbook, from a largely European perspective.]

Sparrow, S. P., & Erhardt, D. (2014). *Essentials of ADHD assessment for children and adolescents.* Hoboken, NJ: Wiley. [Clearly written, authoritative guide for evidence-based assessment of ADHD.]

Tung, I., Li, J. J., Meza, J. I., Jezior, K. L., Kianmahd, J. S. V., Hentschel, P. G., . . . Lee, S. S. (2016). Patterns of comorbidity among girls with ADHD: A meta-analysis. *Pediatrics, 138,* e20160430. [Thorough review of the comorbid conditions linked with ADHD.]

Wolraich, M. L., Chan, E., Froelich, T., Lynch, R. L., Bax, A., Redwine, S. T., . . . Hagan, J. F. (2019). ADHD diagnosis and treatment guidelines: A historical perspective. *Pediatrics, 144,* e20191682. [Analysis of how the current guidelines for assessment and treatment of ADHD, from the American Academy of Pediatrics, emerged.]

Youngstrom, E. A., Prinstein, M. J., Mash, E. J., & Barkley, R. A. (Eds.). (2010). *Assessment of disorders in childhood and adolescence* (5th ed.). New York: Guilford Press. [Major edited textbook of assessment strategies for ADHD and a number of additional conditions.]

Chapter 3: What Is the Outlook for Girls with ADHD?

Biederman, J., Petty, C. R., Monuteaux, M. C., Fried, R., Byrne, D., Mirto, T., . . . Faraone, S. V. (2010). Adult psychiatric outcomes of girls with attention deficit hyperactivity disorder: 11-year follow-up in a longitudinal case-control study. *American Journal of Psychiatry, 167,* 409–417. [Key research article on the follow-up of the Massachusetts General Hospital sample of girls with ADHD.]

Fitzgerald, C., Dalsgaard, S., Nordentoft, M., & Erlangsen, A. (2019). Suicidal behaviour among persons with attention deficit hyperactivity disorder. *British Journal of Psychiatry, 215,* 615–620. [Important article on self-harm as related to individuals with ADHD.]

Garas, P., & Balazs, J. (2020). Long-term suicide risk of children and adolescents with attention deficit and hyperactivity disorder: A systematic review. *Frontiers in Psychiatry, 11,* 557909. [Important scholarly review of suicidal behavior as an outcome of youth with ADHD.]

Guelzow, B. T., Loya, F., & Hinshaw, S. P. (2017). How persistent is ADHD into adulthood?: Informant report and diagnostic thresholds in a female sample. *Journal of Abnormal Child Psychology, 45,* 301–312. [Research article from BGALS investigation regarding the long-term persistence of ADHD in girls.]

Guendelman, M., Ahmad, S., Meza, J. I., Owens, E. B., & Hinshaw, S. P. (2016). Childhood attention-deficit/hyperactivity disorder predicts intimate partner victimization in young women. *Journal of Abnormal Child Psychology, 44,* 155–166. [Research article from BGALS investigation revealing that girls with ADHD are at high risk for experiencing victimization from romantic partners as they grow older.]

Guendelman, M., Owens, E. B., Galan, C., Gard, A., & Hinshaw, S. P. (2016). Early adult correlates of maltreatment in girls with ADHD: Increased risk for internalizing problems and suicidality. *Development and Psychopathology, 28,* 1–14. [Research article from BGALS investigation showing that the experience of physical or sexual abuse, or neglect, during childhood substantially raises the risk of suicide attempts in girls with ADHD by early adulthood.]

Hinshaw, S. P., with Kranz, R. (2009). *The triple bind: Saving our teenage girls from today's pressures.* New York: Ballantine/Random House. [Book-length account of the triple-bind hypothesis that is described in the main text of this chapter.]

Hinshaw, S. P., Owens, E. B., Zalecki, C., Huggins, S. P., Montenegro-Nevado, A., Schrodek,

E., & Swanson, E. N. (2012). Prospective follow-up of girls with attention-deficit hyperactivity disorder into young adulthood: Continuing impairment includes elevated risk for suicide attempts and self-injury. *Journal of Consulting and Clinical Psychology, 80,* 1041–1051. [Research article from BGALS investigation detailing high risk for impairment, including self-harm, in girls with ADHD by the earliest years of adulthood.]

Meza. J. I., Owens, E. O., & Hinshaw, S. P. (2020). Childhood predictors and moderators of lifetime risk for self-harm in girls with and without attention deficit hyperactivity disorder. *Development and Psychopathology, 33,* 1351–1367. [Research article from BGALS investigation revealing the childhood factors that predict risk for later self-harm in girls with ADHD.]

Owens, E. B., Zalecki, C., Gillette, P., & Hinshaw, S. P. (2017). Girls with childhood ADHD as adults: Cross-domain outcomes by diagnostic status. *Journal of Consulting and Clinical Psychology, 85,* 723–736. [Research article from BGALS investigation revealing the many domains of impairment experienced by girls with ADHD by their mid-20s.]

Owens, E. B., Zalecki, C., & Hinshaw, S. P. (2017). Longitudinal investigation of girls with ADHD. In L. T. Hechtman (Ed.), *Attention deficit hyperactivity disorder: Adult outcome and its predictors* (pp. 179–229). New York: Oxford University Press. [Chapter providing overview of BGALS investigation.]

Sibley, M. H., Arnold, L. E., Swanson, J. M., Hechtman, L. T., Kennedy, T. M., Owens, E., ... Rohde, L. A. (2022). Variable patterns of remission from ADHD in the Multimodal Treatment Study of ADHD. *American Journal of Psychiatry, 179*(2), 142–151. [Research article on MTA study showing that, for both girls and boys with ADHD, patterns of the persistence of diagnosis wax and wane in adolescence and adulthood but the vast majority of participants retain symptoms and impairments.]

Skoglund, C., Kopp Kallner, H., Skalkidou, A., Wikström, A. K., Lundin, C., Hesselman, S., ... Sundstrom Poromaa, I. (2019). Association of attention-deficit/hyperactivity disorder with teenage birth among women and girls in Sweden. *JAMA Network Open, 2,* e1912463. [European research article documenting that ADHD is a risk factor for high rates of teenage parenting.]

Uchida, M., Spencer, T. J., Faraone, S. V., & Biederman, J. (2018). Adult outcome of ADHD: An overview of results from the MGH longitudinal family studies of pediatrically and psychiatrically referred youth with and without ADHD of both sexes. *Journal of Attention Disorders, 22,* 523–534. [Review article summarizing the many studies of long-term follow-up of both girls and boys with ADHD from the Massachusetts General Hospital samples.]

Chapter 4: What Do You Need to Know about the Causes of ADHD?

Asherson, P., & Agnew-Blais, J. (2019). Does late-onset attention-deficit/hyperactivity disorder exist? *Journal of Child Psychology and Psychiatry, 60,* 333–352. [Important review article showing that the evidence for the sudden emergence of ADHD in adulthood is highly unlikely, although in many cases detection may not occur until adolescence.]

Boyce, W. T. (2019). *The orchid and the dandelion: Why some children struggle and how all can thrive.* New York: Knopf. [Book-length account of the "differential susceptibility" hypothesis that youth with "risky" genotypes may actually thrive with nurturing environments.]

Faraone, S. V., & Larsson, H. (2019). Genetics of attention deficit hyperactivity disorder. *Molecular Psychiatry, 24,* 562–575. [Review article on the large role of genes in relation to ADHD.]

Hinshaw, S. P., & Ellison, K. (2015). *ADHD: What everyone needs to know.* New York: Oxford University Press. [Easy-to-read book on all aspects of ADHD, including causal factors.]

Nigg, J. T. (2006). *What causes ADHD?: Understanding what goes wrong and why.* New York: Guilford Press. [Book-length account of causal forces for ADHD.]

Nigg, J. T., Sibley, M. H., Thapar, A., & Karalunas, S. L. (2020). Development of ADHD: Etiology, heterogeneity, and early life course. *Annual Review of Developmental Psychology, 2,* 559–583. [Excellent review article on the early-life determinants of ADHD.]

Shaw, P., Lerch, J., Greenstein, D., Sharp, W., Clasen, L., Evans, A., . . . Rapoport, J. (2006). Longitudinal mapping of cortical thickness and clinical outcome in children and adolescents with attention-deficit/hyperactivity disorder. *Archives of General Psychiatry, 63,* 540–549. [Original research article of Shaw and NIH colleagues on frontal cortex immaturity in youth with ADHD.]

Shaw, P., Malek, M., Watson, B., Greenstein, D., de Rossi, P., & Sharp, W. (2013). Trajectories of cerebral cortical development in childhood and adolescence and adult attention-deficit/hyperactivity disorder. *Biological Psychiatry, 74,* 599–606. [Research article on follow-up study to Shaw et al. (2006), above, revealing that delayed cortical development in ADHD continues during adolescence and early adulthood.]

Sripada, C. S., Kessler, D., & Angstadt, M. (2014). Lag in maturation of the brain's intrinsic functional architecture in attention-deficit/hyperactivity disorder. *Proceedings of the National Academy of Sciences of the USA.* www.pnas.org/cgi/doi/10.1073/pnas.1407787111. [Research article on the brain connections underlying ADHD, revealing a developmental lag in such connectivity, supplementing the Shaw et al. articles listed above.]

Thapar, A. (2018). Discoveries on the genetics of ADHD in the 21st century: New findings and their implications. *American Journal of Psychiatry, 175,* 943–950. [Academic article on genes in relation to ADHD.]

Chapter 5: Principles for Parenting a Girl with ADHD

Baumrind, D. (2013). Authoritative parenting revisited: History and current status. In R. E. Larzelere, A. S. Morris, & A. W. Harrist (Eds.), *Authoritative parenting: Synthesizing nurturance and discipline for optimal child development* (pp. 11–34). Washington, DC: American Psychological Association. [Chapter-length review of the concept of authoritative parenting.]

Darling, N., & Steinberg, L. (1993). Parenting style as context: An integrative model. *Psychological Bulletin, 113,* 487–496. [Classic review article on the principles of authoritative (and other) parenting styles.]

Deater-Deckard, K., Dodge, K. A., Bates, J. E., & Pettit, G. S. (1996). Physical discipline among African American and European American mothers: Links to children's externalizing behaviors. *Developmental Psychology, 32,* 1065–1072. [Empirical study suggesting strongly that authoritarian parenting is a risk factor for later antisocial behavior in White families but not in Black families.]

Gordon, C. T., & Hinshaw, S. P. (2017). Parenting stress as a mediator between childhood ADHD and early adult female outcomes. *Journal of Clinical Child and Adolescent Psychology, 46,* 588–599. [Research article from BGALS investigation on the importance of parenting stress in predicting negative outcomes in girls with ADHD.]

Harold, G. T., Leve, L. D., Barrett, D., Elam, K., Neiderheiser, J. M., Natsuaki, M. N., . . . Thapar, A. (2013). Biological and rearing mother influences on child ADHD symptoms: Revisiting the developmental interface between nature and nurture. *Journal of Child Psychology and Psychiatry, 54,* 1038–1046. [Research article revealing that parenting by adoptive parents plays a key role in outcomes for children with ADHD.]

Hinshaw, S. P., Zupan, B. A., Simmel, C., Nigg, J. T., & Melnick, C. (1997). Peer status in boys with and without attention-deficit hyperactivity disorder: Predictions from overt and covert antisocial behavior, social isolation, and authoritative parenting beliefs. *Child*

Development, 68, 880–896. [Research article revealing that authoritative parenting beliefs in primary caregivers of boys with ADHD predict socially competent behavior.]

Maccoby, E. E. (1992). The role of parents in the socialization of children: An historical overview. *Developmental Psychology, 28,* 1006–1017. [Classic article on parenting practices and styles, integrating biology and socialization.]

Meza. J. I., Owens, E. O., & Hinshaw, S. P. (2020). Childhood predictors and moderators of lifetime risk for self-harm in girls with and without attention deficit hyperactivity disorder. *Development and Psychopathology, 33,* 1351–1367. [Research article from BGALS investigation revealing the childhood factors that predict risk for later self-harm in girls with ADHD, including negative father–daughter interactions.]

Pettit, G. S., Laird, R. D., Dodge, K. A., Bates, J. E., & Criss, M. M. (2001). Antecedents and behavior-problem outcomes of parental monitoring and psychological control in early adolescence. *Child Development, 72,* 583–598. [Important research article revealing that strong parental monitoring is associated with lower levels of adolescent aggression and antisocial behavior.]

Sellers, R., Harold, G. T., Smith, A. F., Neiderheiser, J. M., Reiss, D., Shaw, D., . . . Leve, L. D. (2021). Disentangling nature from nurture in examining the interplay between parent–child relationships, ADHD, and early academic attainment. *Psychological Medicine, 51,* 645–652. [Following Harold et al. (2013), another key finding from an adoptive sample that parenting really matters for children with ADHD.]

Chapter 6: Core Treatments for ADHD in Childhood and Adolescence

Barkley, R. A. (2022). *Treating ADHD in children and adolescents: What every clinician needs to know.* New York: Guilford Press. [Authoritative guide on multiple aspects of ADHD, written for clinicians but with valuable information for parents. Nearly every chapter deals with treatments, both psychosocial and medication-related.]

Bikic, A., Reichow, B., McCauley, S. A., Ibrahim, K., & Sukhodolsky, D. B. (2017). Meta-analysis of organizational skills interventions for children and adolescents with attention-deficit/hyperactivity disorder. *Clinical Psychology Review, 52,* 108–123. [Review of organizational skills treatments for ADHD.]

Chronis-Tuscano, A., O'Brien, K., & Danko, C. (2021). *Supporting caregivers of children with ADHD.* New York: Oxford University Press. [Book-length treatise on how different kinds of parents/caregivers, including those with mental-health conditions, can help support interventions for their children with ADHD.]

Gallagher, R., Abikoff, H. B., & Spira, E. G. (2014). *Organizational skills training for children with ADHD: An empirically supported treatment.* New York: Guilford Press. [Book-length review of organizational skills treatment for ADHD.]

Kok, F. M., Groen, Y., Fuermaier, A. B., & Tucha, O. (2020). The female side of pharma-cotherapy for ADHD—A systematic literature review. *PLOS ONE, 15,* e0239257. [Review of the responses of females to medication treatments for ADHD, including information that girls may respond better than boys to nonstimulant medications.]

Kollins, S. H., DeLoss, D. J., Canadas, E., Lutz, J., Findling, R. L., Keefe, R. S. E., . . . Faraone, S. V. (2020). A novel digital intervention for actively reducing severity of paediatric ADHD (STARS-ADHD): A randomised controlled trial. *Lancet Digital Health, 2,* e168–e178. [Research article on interactive video game designed to improve core symptoms of ADHD.]

Mikami, A. Y. (2015). Social skills training for youth with ADHD. In R. A. Barkley (Ed.), *Attention deficit hyperactivity disorder: A handbook for diagnosis and treatment* (4th ed., pp. 569–595). New York: Guilford Press. [Important chapter on the ways in which social skills interventions for youth with ADHD can and do work effectively.]

Moore, D. A., Richardson, M., Gwernan-Jones, R., Thompson-Coon, J., Stein, K., Rogers, M., . . . Ford, T. J. (2019). Non-pharmacological interventions for ADHD in school settings: An overarching synthesis of systematic reviews. *Journal of Attention Disorders, 23,* 220–233. [Review of a variety of psychosocial and psychoeducational interventions for students with ADHD in school settings.]

Nigg, J. T. (2017). *Getting ahead of ADHD: What next-generation science says about treatments that work—and how you can make them work for your child.* New York: Guilford Press. [Book-length review of evidence-based treatments for ADHD, including valuable information on a range of additional treatment modalities.]

Pfiffner, L. J., Dvorsky, M., & Kaiser, N. (2021). Behavioral parent training. In M. K. Dulcan (Ed.), *The American Psychiatric Publishing, Inc. (AAPI) textbook of child and adolescent psychiatry* (3rd ed.). Washington, DC: American Psychiatric Association. [Chapter-length review of behavioral family therapy for ADHD.]

Pfiffner, L. J., Hinshaw, S. P., Owens, E. B., Zalecki, C., Kaiser, N., Villodas, M., & McBurnett, K. (2014). A two-site randomized clinical trial of integrated psychosocial treatment for ADHD–Inattentive type. *Journal of Consulting and Clinical Psychology, 82,* 1115–1127. [Research article showing the effectiveness of the Child Life and Attention Skills (CLAS) intervention for children with the inattentive presentation of ADHD.]

Spence, S. H., O'Shea, G., & Donovan, C. L. (2016). Improvements in interpersonal functioning following interpersonal psychotherapy (IPT) with adolescents and their association with change in depression. *Behavioural and Cognitive Psychotherapy, 44,* 257–272. [Research article documenting improvements in social functioning and depression for adolescents with depression during and after IPT.]

Chapter 7: Educating Your Daughter with ADHD

Arnold, L. E. (2021). Editorial: An inconvenient finding: School accommodations for attention-deficit/hyperactivity disorder. *Journal of the American Academy of Child and Adolescent Psychiatry, 60,* 435–437. [Commentary on the Lovett and Nelson article, below, on the lack of evidence for effectiveness of many accommodations for school-children with ADHD.]

Barkley, R. A. (2016). *Managing ADHD in school: The best evidence-based methods for teachers.* Eau Claire, WI: Pesi Publishing and Media. [Brief but timely handbook on educational interventions and tips for managing ADHD in school settings.]

Becker, S. P. (Ed.). (2020). *ADHD in adolescents: Development, assessment, and treatment.* New York: Guilford Press. [Edited book with excellent range of chapters on ADHD during the teen years. See especially Chapters 8, 13, 14, 15, 16, 17, and 18.]

Harrison, J. R., Bunford, N., Evans, S. W., & Owens, J. S. (2013). Educational accommodations for students with behavioral challenges: A systematic review of the literature. *Review of Educational Research, 83,* 551–597. [Review of effects of educational accommodations for students with a range of behavioral and learning issues.]

Harrison, J. R., Soares, D. A., Rudzinski, S., & Johnson, R. (2019). Attention deficit hyperactivity disorders and classroom-based interventions: Evidence-based status, effectiveness, and moderators of effects in single-case design research. *Review of Educational Research, 89,* 569–611. [Review article on classroom interventions for students with ADHD, from experimental single-case designs, revealing evidence for effectiveness.]

Hart, K. C., Massetti, G. M., Fabiano, G. A., Pariseau, M. E., & Pelham, W. E. (2011). Impact of group size on classroom on-task behavior and work productivity in children with ADHD. *Journal of Emotional and Behavioral Disorders, 19,* 55–64. [Research study revealing that children with ADHD are more on-task during small-group than large-group or individual seatwork instructional conditions.]

Lovett, B. J., & Nelson, J. M. (2021). Systematic review: Educational accommodations for children and adolescents with attention-deficit/hyperactivity disorder. *Journal of the American Academy of Child and Adolescent Psychiatry, 60,* 448–457. [Review article revealing that many school-based accommodations for youth with ADHD have little or no research evidence for effectiveness.]

Pfiffner, L. J. (2011). *All about ADHD: The complete practical guide for classroom teachers* (2nd ed.). New York: Scholastic. [Readable and extremely practical book designed for classroom teachers—and parents—of children with ADHD, through eighth grade.]

Singh, I. (2008). ADHD, culture, and education. *Early Child Development and Care, 178,* 347–361. [Article revealing the social and historical context of schooling in the United States and how a given culture's tolerance for behavioral differences can contextualize treatment and education practices related to ADHD.]

Stanberry, K., & Raskind, M. (2020). Assistive technology for ADHD challenges at school. *ADDitude Magazine, https://additudemag.com/change-the-program*

Chapter 8: Helping Your Young Daughter with ADHD Thrive

Blachman, D. R., & Hinshaw, S. P. (2002).Patterns of friendship in girls with and without attention-deficit/hyperactivity disorder. *Journal of Abnormal Child Psychology, 30,* 625–640. [Research article from BGALS investigation revealing that it's harder for girls with ADHD to make friends or have nonconflictual relationships with friends than it is for typical girls.]

Campbell, S. B. (2007). *Behavior problems in preschool children: Clinical and developmental issues* (2nd ed.). New York: Guilford Press. [Book-length compendium of real wisdom about how to assess and treat behavior problems, including ADHD, in young children.]

Cardoos, S., & Hinshaw, S. P. (2011). Friendship as protection from peer victimization for girls with and without ADHD. *Journal of Abnormal Child Psychology, 39,* 1035–1045. [Research article from BGALS investigation revealing that at least one good-quality friendship can help girls with ADHD from being victimized by peers.]

Caye, A., Petresco, S., de Barros, A. J. D., Bressan, R. A., Gadelha, A., Goncalves, H., . . . Rohde, L. A. (2020). Relative age and attention-deficit/hyperactivity disorder: Data from three epidemiological cohorts and a meta-analysis. *Journal of the American Academy of Child & Adolescent Psychiatry, 59,* 990–997. [Research article and review revealing that being young at kindergarten placement is in fact associated with subsequent risk for diagnosis of ADHD, not always due to misdiagnosis.]

Dadds, M. R., & Tully, L. A. (2019). What is it to discipline a child: What should it be?: A reanalysis of time-out from the perspective of child mental health, attachment, and trauma. *American Psychologist, 74,* 794–808. [Provocative and important review article revealing that time-out procedures actually enhance attachment, when performed optimally.]

Gordon, C. T., & Hinshaw, S. P. (2017). Parenting stress as a mediator between childhood ADHD and early adult female outcomes. *Journal of Clinical Child and Adolescent Psychology, 46,* 588–599. [Research article from BGALS investigation on the importance of parenting stress in predicting negative outcomes in girls with ADHD.]

Hartup, W. W. (1996). The company they keep: Friendships and their developmental significance. *Child Development, 67,* 1–13. [Classic article on the importance of good-quality friendships for development.]

Hinshaw, S. P. (2002). Preadolescent girls with attention deficit/hyperactivity disorder: I. Background characteristics, comorbidity, cognitive and social functioning, and parenting practices. *Journal of Consulting and Clinical Psychology, 70,* 1086–1098. [Research article documenting the many areas of impairment experienced by girls with ADHD during childhood.]

Meza. J. I., Owens, E. O., & Hinshaw, S. P. (2020). Childhood predictors and moderators of lifetime risk for self-harm in girls with and without attention deficit hyperactivity disorder. *Development and Psychopathology, 33,* 1351–1367. [Research article from BGALS investigation on the childhood risk factors for later impairments in girls with ADHD.]

Mikami, A. Y. (2015). Social skills training for youth with ADHD. In R. A. Barkley (Ed.), *Attention deficit hyperactivity disorder: A handbook for diagnosis and treatment* (4th ed., pp. 569–595). New York: Guilford Press. [Important chapter on the ways in which social skills interventions for youth with ADHD can and do work effectively.]

Smit, S., Mikami, A. Y., & Normand, S. (2021). Effects of the Parental Friendship Coaching intervention on parental emotion socialization of children with ADHD. *Research on Child and Adolescent Psychopathology, 50,* 101–115. [Research article revealing that structured parental coaching intervention can have benefits on children with ADHD.]

Wilens, T. E., & Hammerness, P. G. (2016). *Straight talk about psychiatric medications for kids* (4th ed.). New York: Guilford Press. [Authoritative book on medications for youth with mental and neurodevelopmental disorders, including ADHD.]

Chapter 9: Helping Your Teenage Daughter with ADHD Thrive

Antshel, K. M., Faraone, S. V., & Gordon, M. (2014). Cognitive-behavioral treatment outcomes of adolescent ADHD. *Journal of Attention Disorders, 18,* 483–495. [Research article revealing positive outcomes of treatment of teens with ADHD via CBT, particularly those with comorbid anxiety or depression.]

Becker, S. P. (Ed.). (2020). *ADHD in adolescents: Development, assessment, and treatment.* New York: Guilford Press. [Edited book with excellent range of chapters on ADHD during the teen years. See especially Chapters 8, 13, 14, 17, and 18. For information about CHP-AS and HOPS, as described in the chapter text, see Chapter 15 by Langberg et al. For CBT-related information, as described in the chapter text, see Chapter 16 by Sprich and Burbridge.]

Caye, A., Spaldini, A. V., Karam, R. G., Grevet, E., J., Rovaris, D. L., Cau, C. H., . . . Kieling, C. (2016). Predictors of persistence of ADHD into adulthood: A systematic review of the literature and meta-analysis. *European Child and Adolescent Psychiatry, 25,* 1151–1159. [Review article revealing that severity of ADHD, along with comorbid conduct disorder and comorbid depression, were predictors of the persistence of ADHD into adulthood in both boys and girls.]

Fabiano, G. A., Schatz, N. K., Morris, K. L., Willoughby, M. T., Vujnovik, R. K., Hulme, K. F., . . . Pelham, W. E. (2016). Efficacy of a family-focused intervention for young drivers with attention-deficit hyperactivity disorder. *Journal of Consulting and Clinical Psychology, 84,* 1068–1093. [Research article on a family-based intervention for driving skills for teens with ADHD, revealing some positive effects.]

Guendelman, M., Ahmad, S., Meza, J. I., Owens, E. B., & Hinshaw, S. P. (2016). Childhood attention-deficit/hyperactivity disorder predicts intimate partner victimization in young women. *Journal of Abnormal Child Psychology, 44,* 155–166. [Research article from BGALS investigation on the risk for experiencing dating violence/victimization in girls with ADHD by adolescence and young adulthood.]

Hinshaw, S. P., with Kranz, R. (2009). *The triple bind: Saving our teenage girls from today's pressures.* New York: Ballantine/Random House. [Book-length account of the triple-bind hypothesis described in Chapter 3 and again in Chapter 9.]

Meza, J., Owens, E. B., & Hinshaw, S. P. (2016). Response inhibition, peer preference and victimization, and self-harm: Longitudinal associations in young adult women with and without ADHD. *Journal of Abnormal Child Psychology, 44,* 323–334. [Research article from BGALS investigation revealing that peer bullying/victimization in adolescence mediates the linkage between childhood ADHD and NSSI, whereas peer rejection in adolescence mediates the linkage to attempted suicide.]

Mikami, A. M., Szwedo, D. E., Ahmad, S. I., Samuels, A. S., & Hinshaw, S. P. (2015). Online social communication patterns among young adult women with histories of childhood attention-deficit/hyperactivity disorder. *Journal of Abnormal Psychology, 124,* 576–588. [Research article from BGALS investigation revealing that girls with ADHD tend to "overuse" social media, at the expense of actual peer relationships.]

McGuire, E. A., Kolko, D. J., Joseph, H. M., Kipp, H. L., Kindstrom, R. A., Pederson, S. L., . . . Molina, B. S. G. (2021). Use of stimulant diversion prevention strategies in pediatric primary care and associations with provider characteristics. *Journal of Adolescent Health, 68,* 808–815. [Initial research article on means of preventing the diversion of stimulants from teens with ADHD to their peers by engaging pediatricians.]

Miller, W. R., & Rollnick, S. (2013). *Motivational interviewing: Helping people change* (3rd ed.). New York: Guilford Press. [Book-length account of motivational interviewing, one of the bases of the STAND program as described in the chapter text.]

Owens, E. B., & Hinshaw, S. P. (2020). Adolescent mediators of unplanned pregnancy among young women with and without childhood ADHD. *Journal of Clinical Child and Adolescent Psychology, 49,* 229–238. [Research article from BGALS investigation revealing that poor academic performance in adolescence mediates the linkage between childhood ADHD and later unplanned pregnancy.]

Settani, M., Marengo, D., Fabris, M. A., & Longobardi, C. (2018). The interplay between ADHD symptoms and time perspective in addictive social media use: A study on adolescent Facebook users. *Child and Youth Services Review, 89,* 165–170. [Research article—not contending that social media use "causes" ADHD but instead that higher levels of ADHD symptoms predict problematic Facebook usage—with implications for negative perceptions of past and present experiences.]

Sibley, M. H. (2017). *Parent–teen therapy for executive function deficits and ADHD: Building skills and motivation.* New York: Guilford Press. [Book-length account of the behavioral and motivational interviewing origins of the STAND program designed by Sibley.]

Sibley, M. H., Altszuler, A. R., Morrow, A. S., & Merrill, B. M. (2014). Mapping the academic problem behaviors of adolescents with ADHD. *School Psychology Quarterly, 29,* 422–437. [Article on the Adolescent Academic Problems Checklist, a rating instrument for parents, teachers, and teens to appraise the range of experienced academic problems.]

Swanson, E. N., Owens, E. B., & Hinshaw, S. P. (2014). Pathways to self-harmful behaviors in young women with and without ADHD: A longitudinal examination of mediating factors. *Journal of Child Psychology and Psychiatry, 55,* 505–515. [Research article from BGALS investigation revealing that poor executive functions and externalizing behavior in adolescence mediate the linkage between childhood ADHD and NSSI, whereas adolescent internalizing behaviors mediate the link to later suicidal behavior.]

Chapter 10: Looking Ahead

Dvorsky, M. R., & Langberg, J. M. (2016). A review of factors that promote resilience in youth with ADHD and ADHD symptoms. *Clinical Child and Family Psychology Review, 19,* 368–391. [Review of the studies that examine protective factors for kids with ADHD between childhood and later-life outcomes.]

Hinshaw, S. P. (2018). Attention deficit hyperactivity disorder (ADHD): Controversy, developmental mechanisms, and multiple levels of analysis. *Annual Review of Clinical Psychology, 14,* 291–316. [Review article featuring information on many aspects of ADHD.]

Hinshaw, S. P., Nguyen, N. T., O'Grady, S. M., & Rosenthal, E. A. (2022). ADHD in girls and women: Underrepresentation, longitudinal processes, and key directions. *Journal of Child Psychology and Psychiatry, Annual Research Review, 63,* 484–496. [Review of historical trends related to underrecognition of ADHD in girls and women, as well as accumulated research on girls and women with ADHD and prospects for future research.]

Hinshaw, S. P., & Scheffler, R. M. (2014). *The ADHD explosion: Myths, medication, money, and today's push for performance.* New York: Oxford University Press. [Comprehensive book on controversies related to ADHD, myths and realities of ADHD, and influence of state-by-state testing policies on greatly differing rates of ADHD diagnoses within the United States.]

Martinez, A., & Hinshaw, S. P. (2016). Mental health stigma: Theory, developmental issues, and research priorities. In D. Cicchetti (Ed.), *Developmental psychopathology: Vol 4. Risk, resilience, and intervention* (3rd ed., pp. 997–1039). Hoboken, NJ: Wiley. [Lengthy book chapter on multiple aspects of the stigmatization of mental disorders.]

Mowlem, F., Agnew-Blais, J., Taylor, E., & Asherson, P. (2019). Do different factors influence whether girls versus boys meet ADHD diagnostic criteria?: Sex differences among children with high ADHD symptoms. *Psychiatry Research, 272,* 765–773. [Article on factors that may predict underdiagnosis of ADHD in girls, including parental perceptions.]

National Institute for Health and Care Excellence. (2019). *Attention deficit hyperactivity disorder: Diagnosis and management.* Available from *www.nice.org.uk/guidance/ng87.* [Authoritative guide from the United Kingdom on assessment and diagnosis of ADHD.]

Nguyen, P. T., & Hinshaw, S. P. (2020). Understanding the stigma associated with ADHD: Hope for the future? *ADHD Report, 28,* 1–10. [Review article on reasons for and consequences of stigma for individuals with ADHD.]

Pelham, W. E., Foster, E. M., & Robb, J. A. (2007). The economic impact of attention-deficit/hyperactivity disorder in children and adolescents. *Journal of Pediatric Psychology, 32,* 711–727. [Research article revealing the large economic burden associated with ADHD in childhood and adolescence.]

Polanczyk, G. V., Willcutt, E. G., Salum, G. A., Kieling, C., & Rohde, L. A. (2014). ADHD prevalence estimates across three decades: An updated systematic review and meta-regression analysis. *International Journal of Epidemiology, 43,* 434–442. [Review of international research revealing remarkably consistent rates of the prevalence of ADHD around the world.]

Young, S., Adamo, N., Asgeirsdottir, B. B., Branney, P., Beckett, M., Colley, W., . . . Woodhouse, E. (2020). Females with ADHD: An expert consensus statement taking a lifespan approach providing guidance for the identification and treatment of attention-deficit/hyperactivity disorder in girls and women. *BMC Psychiatry, 20,* 404. [Authoritative British review article on manifestations of ADHD in girls and women.]

Index

About the Author

Stephen P. Hinshaw, PhD, is Distinguished Professor of Psychology at the University of California, Berkeley. He is also Professor of Psychiatry and Behavioral Sciences and Vice-Chair for Child and Adolescent Psychology at the University of California, San Francisco. An internationally known ADHD and stigma researcher and the author of numerous articles and books for scientists, professionals, and general readers, Dr. Hinshaw has received, among other awards, the Distinguished Scientific Contributions Award from the American Psychological Association and the Sarnat International Prize in Mental Health from the National Academy of Medicine. He was recently inducted into the American Academy of Arts and Sciences.